THE SEVEN
DISCIPLINES
OF WELLNESS

The Spiritual Connection to Good Health

Surina Ann Jordan, Ph.D.

To The Pages
Thanks for your
witness

Love,

Sis Surina
443-690-7365

Surina Jordan

This book is dedicated to the great *I Am,*
the Source of my existence.

By the same author

◆◆◆

Got Cancer? Congratulations! Now You Can Start Living

Living Well: A Series of Short Articles for Holistic Living

✦✦✦ Contents ✦✦✦

Foreword 6

Introduction 9

Our Struggle for Wellness: The War 11

Wellness Is a Lifestyle 15

The Battle for Wellness 23

The Wellness Battle Plan 29

Discipline 1: Pursue Primary Care 55

Discipline 2: Maintain Good Communication 68

Discipline 3: Be Intentional About Life 82

Discipline 4: Use Common Sense 89

Discipline 5: Establish a Sacred Place to Live 93

Discipline 6: Move 108

Discipline 7: Eat and Drink Real Food 114

The Soldier's Advance 142

Conclusion: The Catalyst for Wellness 146

Recap of the Disciplines 149

Appendix A: Prayers for a Wellness Lifestyle 150

Appendix B: Time Log 152

Appendix C: Natural Household Cleaners 154

Appendix D: Sources of Calcium 155

Appendix E: Weekly Food Planner 156

Bibliography 157

Index 164

Acknowledgements 170

FOREWORD

S urina Ann Jordan's *The Seven Disciplines of Wellness* is a comprehensive tour de force through the world of wellness, balanced in its survey of the social, spiritual, emotional and physical barriers to an individual's achievement of wellness. Surina lays the foundation by introducing her readers to a concept of wellness as "unbroken completeness" of the three components of man: body, mind, and spirit. Each of the components of this "trinity of man" requires attention when moving away from what she calls the "diseased culture" to a lifestyle of wellness. At the core of her discourse is the proclamation that it is necessary for anyone on the quest to completeness to recognize God as the source of life from which all else flows. Like Adam, possession of free will enables us to choose to break free from a culture wrought with impediments to health, such as processed foods, targeted marketing of unhealthy products, and busy lives reflecting poor stewardship of our time and resources when it comes to our own wellness. The choice to place God as priority in all that we do is the author's cry throughout *The Seven Disciplines of Wellness*.

Her approach to achieving wellness is both spiritual and cerebral without losing sight of the practical applications of the concepts she presents. The reader will become empowered to incorporate life-changing, sustainable practices which will permeate every aspect of her life. The reader will learn to apply the disciplines of pursuing primary care, maintaining good communication, being intentional about life (living on purpose), using common sense, establishing a sacred place to live, and moving (or exercising), in addition to consuming healthy foods.

This book's strengths lie in both its depth of Scripture and its scientific citations to support the principles offered. The author's own lifestyle is a superb example of the genuine embodiment of the Seven Disciplines. I have been fortunate to receive advice from Surina on the proper use of vitamins and herbal remedies while traveling together on the missionary field in Lesotho, South Africa. Her insight and passion about nutrition in her community and globally are refreshing and stem from a life completely immersed in holistic living.

Surina's charge to readers to consider the sacredness of their living spaces when configuring a wellness-supportive home environment is a special jewel, among many, in this insightful book. As myself a physician in the field of Internal Medicine and a minister of the faith, I believe Surina has successfully consummated the relationship between science and spirituality with this book. People of faith will, of course, connect readily to the concepts presented herein, while others will be drawn by the philosophical and scientific information presented. The common sense and wellness thought points in each section, and the tables covering a myriad of wellness lifestyle concepts, are great references that make this a resource to be utilized long after one's initial reading.

Cozzette Lyons-Jones, M.D.
Los Angeles, CA

INTRODUCTION

I have been a wellness teacher, practitioner, and counselor in Christian communities across the United States for 20 years. Within that time, I have noticed that when it comes to health and wellness for Christians today, the most significant problem is that they have not made the connection between their relationship with Christ and their health. Wellness has a spiritual underpinning. When the children of God understand this, they gain the motivation needed to change and become healthier. Being healthy becomes a part of good stewardship, and good stewardship requires discipline.

Individuals who want to live healthier lives, prevent disease, strengthen their walk with God, and help family and friends become or remain healthy should read this book. Reading this book simplifies how to improve your health by removing the noise of the health and wellness industries and gives you a clear focus of health and wellness on God's terms.

I believe that a person cannot experience whole health without a relationship with God through Jesus Christ. On our own, we can never be well. I want to help synthesize all the health information available. I have created a path with seven easy-to-remember disciplines for becoming healthier.

These disciplines are designed to educate you consciously. However, the effectiveness of these disciplines will plant seeds of change that will hopefully resonate at the subconscious level, taking root within your value system and providing the motivation to change behavior in your daily struggle to be well. For the purposes of this book, I will use the terms health, well, and wellness interchangeably. These terms not only mean the absence of disease, but they also refer to an overall sense of mental, spiritual and physical well-being.

When you have completed this book, you will understand what health is on God's terms, the nature of disease, and how to reduce the chances of disease. You can get started on these simple steps immediately and recognize the positive changes in your life. You will know the Seven Disciplines that bring about better health and why they are important.

As humans, we naturally assume that our health is one of our greatest assets, and it's true. Believe me when I say that no matter how bad your health is, you can recover, even from something as devastating as cancer (I write about this in my other book *Got Cancer? Congratulations! Now You Can Start Living*). I, and people close to me, have experienced poor health. With the Seven Disciplines, we were able to turn our lives around, and so can you!

Why do we need the Seven Disciplines? Experts in a field (e.g., sports, medicine, education) have a set of habits and disciplines that yield success. Scripture clearly tells Christians that living for Christ is not always easy. It can sometimes feel like we are soldiers in a war. If you plan to stay in the fight, you must be fit. We must know and understand the tools that have been given to us in order to fight the many battles that occur over a lifetime. All of this requires a consistent way of doing things that have been proven to stand the test of time and yield expected results. If we want to be well and remain well regardless of age, **we need discipline**.

In certain chapters, I have included a common sense conclusion and a wellness thought to provide you with a take away lesson.

 A common sense conclusion.

 Wellness thought.

OUR STRUGGLE FOR WELLNESS: THE WAR

M ost wars don't make a lot of sense. Discussion resolves most issues if the parties involved understand and agree to an outcome for the greater good. However, this does not make the act of war less serious. Wars are devastating. The war that has been going on before we were born is the fight against an evil presence in the universe that seeks to destroy all of God's creation. From nature to populations, this evil presence schemes to destroy all! The battle against the health and well-being of people is very serious. It is part of the overall strategy to destroy God's most valued creation. Many of us see the devastation but have never viewed it in the context of a war. As a result, we don't become engaged enough to fight the opposition and survive. The battle for good health is not fought with bullets, guns, or missiles; it is subtler than that. The weapon the evil force uses in this battle is a culture that redefines truth, values, and language. This culture creates a way of doing things that results in sickness, pain, and premature death. Wars leave behind devastation. The Book of Revelation clearly indicates who wins this war: God through Jesus Christ.

This war zone is what I call a **diseased culture**. My definition of a diseased culture is one where we embrace a lifestyle that accepts sickness, disease, and dysfunction. It is rebellious by nature. As a result, technology, medicine, culture, commerce, and economics are used to help us live life after we have acquired a disease or support us as we die prematurely from the disease or treatment. A diseased culture is the same as popular culture, "this world," or "this present age," as mentioned in Scripture. It is a culture that has no regard for the things of God and looks to the superficial for direction and solutions to all of the challenges in life.

Evidence of the diseased culture is everywhere. According to the Nutritional Vital Statistics provided by the Centers for Disease Control and Prevention (CDC) in Atlanta, the six leading chronic diseases in the United States include heart disease, cancer, stroke, high blood pressure, chronic obstructive pulmonary disease, and diabetes. In 34 percent of American adults ages 20 and older, these conditions are responsible for 70 percent of the deaths that occur in the U.S. every year.

There are certain underlying elements that perpetuate a diseased culture as a way of life. A primary element is the belief that truth is relative; either there is no truth or the truth keeps changing. With television and the Internet, anyone can become an overnight authority on just about anything. Before, we would seek information from our community, but now we seek information from social media and search engines. We can now have hundreds of friends without leaving our home. As lack of time and individual isolation increase, social media plays into the human need to be in relationships and theoretically reduces the time needed to do so. These digital pen pals often rank high in importance and usually their advice is valued.

Another example of changing truth: we were once told that vitamin C was good for us as proven by chemist and Nobel Prize winner John C. Pauling. Shortly after that, some physicians suggested that vitamin C might not be good for you because it could cause diarrhea and kidney stones. This type of information without supporting evidence leads to confusion. It appears that whoever has the best delivery has the truth, and since the delivery changes so rapidly, confusion and frustration support apathy within the diseased culture.

With each new truth comes a host of companies ready with a "solution" to the problems associated with the disease and sickness. These companies make large profits: $500 billion in 2007. According to Paul Zane Pilzer, economist and author of *The New Wellness Revolution*, "Opportunity for business development and growth will continue well into the next decade" as consumer demand increases. The growth of these companies and their increasing revenue make it difficult to combat them in this diseased culture. It is a struggle, but not impossible, to change this situation.

One of the difficulties with changing the diseased culture is that it is self-sustaining. There is a complex interdependency of organizational behaviors that influence our health. Big businesses shape public policy by lobbying for their cause. Government is buckling under the burden of debt and our leaders are buckling under the fear of not being reelected. Public health organizations lack the resources and leadership to collect and mine data for root causes and prevention methods. Community groups and nonprofits are forced to chase money to stay afloat instead of driving their causes. Researchers are left to support the interests of their grantors, which most often are big businesses or the government. Few universities fund their own research. As a result, research is powered by special interests. Change seems more possible from the consumer.

Another hurdle preventing changing to a wellness culture is many of us have been sedated by popular culture and no longer think or question things. This makes us more vulnerable and easily influenced by the systemic dysfunction.

As consumers, we can expedite change within these and other industries, including the medical, agriculture, food and beverage, and pharmaceutical industries. Within the discussion about health care, prevention, and wellness, an underlying message seems to blame the individual for not taking personal responsibility for his or her health and well-being. From the health department to the hospital, intervention appears one-sided. If the health industry evaluated its role in an individual's struggle to make lasting behavioral change and transitioned to a responsible and sustainable business model, we could move rapidly toward a wellness culture. This industry will respond when we use our purchasing power as our voice. For example, let's look at our willingness to join store memberships and clubs for discounts on products. Yes, consumers reap benefits, but merchants collect data on the buying behaviors and product preferences of their members. Until more consumers change their spending habits and buy products that contribute to their health, the data being collected and passed on to product manufacturers indicates that the same unhealthy products are just fine!

In the meantime, we must use common sense in order to survive. From this discussion, we can see that having a diseased lifestyle is not entirely our fault. Companies have not made it easy to move toward wellness. There is a pharmaceutical preparation for every symptom. Eating well is more costly. Junk food is cheap and more accessible. You can also see that we cannot just go with the flow and expect not to have a health challenge. Wellness will require some simple changes and key decisions as we move forward.

 Good health requires personal involvement on many levels.

 I need to think about how the diseased culture affects me.

WELLNESS
IS A
LIFESTYLE

A wellness lifestyle does not mean that you will never be sick. Wellness is defined as unbroken completeness. It is the health of the mind, body, and spirit. A wellness lifestyle means that the mind (one's intellect and emotion), the body (a person's physical being), and spirit (will and connectedness to God) are in complete harmony.

A wellness lifestyle has, at the very core, the expectation of being well. It does not entertain beliefs, such as "I will be sick because everyone else is sick," "My disease is inevitable due to my family history," "As I age, I will become sick," or that allergies are normal. What a wellness lifestyle does mean is that good stewardship of our personal trinity (mind, body, and spirit) is in place and we have the habit of being well.

Wellness is a common sense way of living. An example of not using common sense would be baby John's parents leaving home without John's meal or diaper bag. Since infants eat frequently with limited options, having their food handy is necessary, with a diaper change being inevitable. **Common sense**, then, is making planned, rational decisions based on what we know to be true. We'll explore using common sense for a healthy lifestyle in Discipline 4.

How we live every day affects the quality of our health and energy levels. Daily investments are needed in order to preserve and protect our bodies from disease and ailments that rob us of quality living. What if you already have a chronic disease? Can wellness still be a lifestyle? Yes, you *can* be well. Your goal for wellness will be to stabilize your condition and reverse and prevent the advancement of the disease while minimizing the side effects of treatment. Preventing the onset of a second chronic disease is also important. For example, high blood pressure and diabetes oftentimes co-exist.

Many of us have never looked at what we do every day and labeled it a lifestyle. However, what we do, what we think, where and with whom we spend our time, and how we spend our resources is, in fact, our lifestyle. Scripture tells us that we should **"never walk away from common sense and clear thinking"** (Proverbs 3:21-26)—things essential to maintaining a wellness lifestyle.

 Wellness is a lifestyle.

Every day, I help keep myself well.

The foundation for wellness is based upon love as a belief system. This belief system is that firm foundation that makes everything about our lives possible and meaningful. God is love (I John 4:8). We must believe that God is all-powerful, all-knowing, and in all places. We must never forget that God made the world and everything in it. He makes the creatures; the creatures don't make Him. Starting from scratch, He made the entire human race and made the earth hospitable.

One of the things we must come to realize is that God (our Manufacturer, if you will) knows His product, His reflection. He built memory chips and routines that maintain our body parts and the internal systems that connect all of those parts. He also put within each of us a feeling of sensitivity to His love. Common sense is one of those built-in features that comes with human life. The ability to decide and make choices is also included. We may choose to live in harmony with God or attempt to live life without Him. A relationship with God is essential for wellness and our ability to care for others and ourselves. We have a feeling of sensitivity to His presence, which provides a sense of safety, well-being, and courage.

Catherine Ponder, author of *The Dynamic Laws of Healing* states, "Choosing life without the spirit of the Creator is the root of all sickness and disease." God is the lover of all we are and all we can become. Bottom line: if you are living life where you have positioned yourself or some other person or thing as a god in your life, then you have a counterfeit god. When we embrace God, we are postured to accomplish our life's purpose and to know wellness. Love stabilizes all other dimensions in life. We are created to live in wellness so the spirit, mind, and body can remain whole.

 Common sense and choice are gifts from God our Creator.

 Wellness is possible because of love.

Knowing God

According to Scripture, God is one being made up of three distinct persons who exist in co-equal, co-eternal communion as the Father, Son, and Holy Spirit. This communion is also known as the Trinity.

God's desire to reflect His nature led to the creation of man and woman. The Book of Genesis (1:26-27) records that God spoke: "Let us make human beings in our image, make them reflecting our nature, so they can be responsible for the Earth itself, and every animal that moves on the face of Earth. God created human beings; He created them godlike, reflecting God's nature. He created them male and female." Man also has three distinct attributes that make up a whole person:

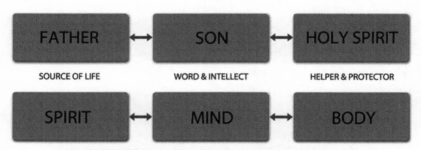

MAN'S PERSONAL TRINITY IN THE IMAGE OF GOD

Each attribute of God and man has a specific role, which represents an essential function. These roles lead to our ability to live well and with purpose. The **Spirit** or the **Father** represents the source of life and the leadership of the whole person. Our spirit is the source of values and

17

character, security, and well-being. The **Son**, Jesus, is the Word and the Intelligence of God. Our minds are wired to that intelligence. The Son, as we will discuss later, is the bridge that allows us access to God. The **Holy Spirit** is the helper, executor, and protector to carry forth the will and mind of the Father and the Son. Our body's activity and senses reflect this.

When man was created, God gave him the power to make choices. This is one of the major attributes that separate humans from animals. God encouraged choice by having man name the animals and other things, as well as manage resources. He provided the path that made our relationship with Him pure and straightforward. God also provided the framework for successful living. He was to be our constant companion and provider. We broke our relationship with Him by stepping outside of that framework. God's enemy, Satan, convinced both man and woman to dishonor God in an attempt to steal God's most precious creation (humans). Satan appealed to Eve's mind, body, and spirit. He successfully tempted her with the fruit from the tree of knowledge, opening her eyes to good and evil. Adam and Eve exercised their gift of choice, which was the beginning of the deterioration of humanity. It meant spiritual death and life apart from God (Genesis 2:16-17). The parameters for survival and abundant living were removed and the battle for wellness began.

We have been wired by God to have Him as our main power source as we navigate through life. It is our sense of well-being and knowing deep within that we are part of a larger picture. It is the desire to know and to be known. It is the need to feel connected, to be valued, and to become a contributor for the common good.

In the 1980s, Burt Bacharach partnered with singer Dionne Warwick to perform his song, "What the World Needs Now Is Love." It goes on to say "it's the only thing that there's just too little of." Unfortunately, the diseased culture often changes the definition of love to be synonymous with lust, gifts, and related emotions. To know love is to know God. Man cannot live without love. And when we try, we begin losing the battle of good health, for God is love. Diane Peters Mayer, a leading psychotherapist says, "This relationship can give you inspiration, peace of mind, the feeling of joyfulness, and a deep satisfaction in knowing that there's direction you can count on."

Wellness is common sense. Common sense is only possible where there is truth. God is also truth. In truth, we discover health, love, life, and the ability to become whole. All other approaches yield partial but vulnerable health conditions, and superficial joy and excitement. However, a wellness lifestyle requires a sense of peace at the very foundation of life. Peace is a tangible benefit of love. Even when hard times come, this peace remains.

Common sense should help us believe in God, and we should also realize that we need God. We must have a relationship with God. As we mature in our relationship with Him, we will see that God is a proper noun and a verb. He *is* and He *does*.

Allow me to give you an account of love in action. God does not acknowledge relationships that are not based on truth and love. By giving us the gift of choice, God saw our potential for wrongdoing from the beginning of time based on how we would use this gift. As time went on, God executed His strategy for getting us back into relationship with Him. He did this by taking on a human form so He could experience our humanity and represent us as the one to pay for all our wrongdoing (sin). That is the evidence-based story of Jesus the Christ (Messiah), the human part of God. Without cause, he was sentenced to death by crucifixion. He died on a cross, which was payment for our sin. He rose from the dead, which made provisions for all people—past, present, and future—to be able to have a relationship with him forever. And with that provision, God reinforced the wiring of us to Himself in the person of His spirit, which assists us with the truth and gives guidance for living on purpose to the end. All we have to do is accept it. The payment even covers our future errors. This strategy was fully executed and successfully completed. The only project that is still being implemented is the offering of that renewed relationship with God to everyone. Jesus did the hard part. In the Book of Isaiah 53:5 we read:

> "But the fact is, it was *our* pains he carried—*our* disfigurements, all the
> things wrong with *us*. We thought he brought it on himself, that God

was punishing him for his own failures. But it was our sins that did that to him, that ripped and tore and crushed him—*our* sins! He took the punishment, and that made us whole. Through his bruises we get healed. We're all like sheep that've wandered off and gotten lost. We've all done our own thing, gone our own way. And God has piled all our sins, everything we've done wrong, on him [Jesus], on him." God desires to have a close personal relationship with each of us. And he never took that gift of choice back from us in the process. The choice to accept Christ or not is still ours to make. If you would like to accept that renewed relationship with God, simply say, *"God, I have been wrong in not living for you. I ask for forgiveness and receive Jesus and your love into my heart now. Thanks. Amen."*

Congratulations! You now have a clean slate to receive the relationship with God that was meant for you from the beginning. You are a part of the Kingdom of God, which is the culture outside of the diseased culture. "I will be a Father to you, and you will be my sons and daughters, says the Lord Almighty" (II Corinthians 6:18, NIV). This provides us with the ability to call God "Father," which is an indication of His role, authority, and love for us. The names of God indicate His blessings and benefits, His power and manner, how He is to be honored, and how He is to be worshiped. Scripture tells us that we should "love the Lord thy God with all thy heart, and with all thy soul, and with all thy mind" (Matthew 22:37, KJV). Jesus the Christ will assist us with knowing how to love God. As you pursue his path, wellness is realized.

So we say praises to the Christ! We thank him and honor him for repairing that broken relationship with God for us. "One man died for everyone. That puts everyone in the same boat. He included everyone in his death so that everyone could also be included in his life, a resurrection life, a far better life than people ever lived on their own" (II Corinthians 5:14-15). Jesus Christ is our hall pass to gain full access to God and His Kingdom. Jesus brought God's Kingdom to earth, according to Matthew 6:10. We are connected! And now with Christ we can be completely whole. With this expression of love, we have the ability to pursue authentic wellness.

We will not always make the right choice. As long as there are choices, there will be battles. There will be battles of confusion, sickness, and agendas that promote an independent existence outside of the Kingdom of God. However, deep inside each of us is the life force (wiring) that is the center of love and well-being.

> God is our Creator. God is Love. God is Truth.
> Jesus fixed our broken relationship with God.

Then why are so many of us very sick? There is a war going on. Now that we are in Christ, however, our spirit has been renewed. Scripture reads, "Therefore if any man be in Christ, he is a **new creature**: old things are passed away; behold, all things are become **new**" (II Corinthians 5:17, KJV). The old person has passed away. Whenever we attempt to live for Christ outside of His Kingdom, we lose our ability to be well. Every day, better health will be realized as you choose to know and take the path that Christ has provided. This lifestyle is wellness. We live outside of the diseased culture—and inside of the Kingdom of God.

That relationship, made possible through Christ our bridge, is what sustains us and is all that is needed to be well. One of the foundational Scriptures that reinforce this dependency is Matthew 22:37, which states that we are to love God with all of our heart, soul, and mind.

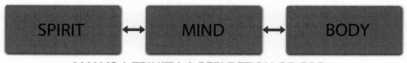

MAN IS A TRINITY, A REFLECTION OF GOD.

Each of us has to make a conscious choice and accept Jesus as Savior. When we accept Christ, we are adopted into God's family and our souls are given life forever. We become a part of His Kingdom. Our goal is to live to glorify God and point others to Christ. So our battle with the enemy Satan is **not** to take our soul; it is no longer up for grabs. The battle is to prevent us from offering Christ to others who are trying to live life without him and to prevent us from fulfilling our life's purpose. **The battleground for wellness is in the mind.** Our choices are between life and death. The thoughts, decisions, and choices that we make keep us in (life) or out of (death) obedience to God. The enemy will try to block our progress by any means necessary.

 Wellness is not possible without God's love and truth.

 I am wired to be well by living outside of the diseased culture and within God's Kingdom.

THE BATTLE FOR WELLNESS

I n order to fight a battle, it is important that we know against whom and what we are fighting. There is a systemic process to destroy humanity. We know that a healthy spirit develops a healthy mind and encourages us to make choices and decisions that are in line with the will and purposes of God. A healthy mind supports a strong body.

We are the most valuable of all creation, empowered to reflect God and His love throughout the world. The enemy of God wages war against us in order to destroy God's prized possessions. The battle is not personal. We are caught in the middle. However, when we give our lives to Christ, he stands in the middle of the fight with us. The enemy of God seeks victory by the destruction of our trinity and by the elimination of the resources needed to sustain our ability to live. As we eat, sleep, move, drink, and live in the way of Christ, the enemy is defeated.

In whom the god [Satan] of this world [culture] hath *blinded the minds* of them which believe not, lest the light of the glorious gospel of Christ, who is the image of God, should shine unto them.
—II Corinthians 4:4 (KJV)

The Enemy's Strategy
Satan's sole strategy is to undo everything God put in place to reflect His nature of love and truth. This strategy of undoing consists of dismantling, destroying, confusing, and breaking our connection to God.

Satan uses anything and anybody to blind our minds to the truth of God's love and our dependency on Him for wellness. The current culture is on autopilot, and messages of truth and authentic wellness have become an aversion to many.

The Destroyer's strategy is to keep us ignorant of our right to make choices and the benefit of choosing God. His weapons are masterful and can destroy your mind. **Our minds are the battlefield.** Satan's goal is to make our decisions, by default, in his ways. But his ways will never reflect God or keep our mind, body, and spirit from destruction. His attacks come from many directions. The enemy uses the media, academia, airwaves, the Internet, religions, marketing, public policies, relationships, and family to infiltrate our lives.

As a result, we live with overloaded minds and emotions. This eventually impacts our spiritual compass, changing values systems, priorities, and relationships. The chemical and hormonal relationship between the mind and brain to the body affects our physical health as well. We must live with a "trinity health" mind-set, understanding that dysfunctional thinking can impact any attribute of our trinity.

Satan celebrates every time he successfully destroys a reflection of God. Here are his major tactics:

- ❖ Make sure that those who are not connected to God stay that way and never know the healing nature of Christ and joy in life.
- ❖ Prevent those who are connected to Christ from bringing others to Christ, and eliminate their ability to bring glory to God the Father.
- ❖ Keep us from remembering that Christ is within us (our renewed mind) so that we will make destructive decisions and choices (our carnal mind).
- ❖ Get us to destroy ourselves through behaviors and thoughts that cause sickness and disease.

A key strategy of the enemy is to destroy the body and confuse the mind. Many Christians are not aware that there is a battle and, as a result, live very defeated lives. Some of us have become our own worst enemy. We have self-destructive behaviors, including negative speech, self-hate, negative thoughts, and disobedience to God's Word.

In order to fight this battle, we must understand the enemy's weapons. Satan has some powerful weapons that have been successful in fighting battles for a long time.

Our minds are the battlefield.

Knowing Your Strengths and Your Weapons

In every battle, we can be confident that Christ is with us and in us. As children of God, we still make mistakes and bad choices; only God is perfect. Whatever the circumstance, as we ask for forgiveness and help, God's love will bring glory out of the situation. *He will keep salvaging our bad choices, and these bad choices are not without consequences, but he will also use them for good.* (Romans 8:28)

You cannot fight the battles for your wellness alone; you will never win on your own. These battles are bigger than you. But know that you are a part of the most powerful army ever. Jesus Christ is our captain and once we have enlisted with him, he will never leave us. He is our Savior.

Christ gives us a spiritual and mental awareness of the power of God within. This awareness, or "Armor of God" as Scripture calls it, is essential for us every day. This awareness leads us toward the wellness path and gives the Holy Spirit full reign to coach us as we live and grow in God's will and purpose for our lives. The Armor of God is outlined in the Book of Ephesians 6:10-18, KJV:

"Finally, my brethren, be strong in the Lord, and in the power of His might. Put on the whole armor of God, that ye may be able to stand against the wiles of the Devil. For we wrestle not against flesh and blood, but against principalities, against powers, against the rulers of the darkness of this world, against spiritual wickedness in high places. Wherefore take unto you the whole armor of God, that ye may be able to withstand in the evil day, and having done all, to stand. Stand therefore, having your loins girt about with truth, and having on the breastplate of **righteousness;** and your feet shod with the preparation of the gospel of **peace;** above all, taking the shield of **faith,** wherewith ye shall be able to quench all the fiery darts of the wicked. And take the helmet of **salvation,** and the sword of the Spirit, which is the **word of God:** praying always with all **prayer** and supplication in the Spirit, and watching thereunto with all perseverance and supplication for all saints."

The protective Armor of God is what we think about to remain at peace in times of trouble and stressful situations. As we study Scripture, we discover that there are many promises God has made to His children:

"I will be your confidence and keep your foot from being taken."
(Proverbs 3:26)
"I know the plans I have for you." (Jeremiah 29:11)
"I will never leave you or forsake you." (Hebrews 13:5)
"Seest thou a man diligent in his business? He shall not stand before mean men." (Proverbs 22:29, KJV)

When we study all of these promises, they will naturally come to mind at the time of need. Sometimes the enemy will throw so much tribulation at us, the pressure can feel like a fire hose. But God said "When the enemy shall come in like a flood, Lord shall lift up a standard against him." (Isaiah 59:19)

God provides the armor but we must put it on.
—Our Daily Bread

The following diagram helps us see how full the Armor of God is, as described in Ephesians 6.

Weapon	Purpose	Our Benefit
Truth	The Holy Spirit, the Spirit of Truth to provide understanding of all things. (John 14:16-17, 26); Freedom (John 8:32)	Common sense; Feeling burden-free; Strength (II Sam. 22:33); Joy (John 15:11); Understanding and help; Less stress, less guilt.
Righteousness	Holy through the blood of Jesus Christ; In right relationship with God; Helps us conform to the will of God (Rom. 12:2).	Life (Rom. 8:10); No baggage; Ability to take the right action.
Peace	Natural state of wholeness; Impact on enemy; Peace wherever we go.	Grounded (Phil. 4:7); Reduces stress; Authentic joy.
Faith	Ability to please God, knowing that He exists; Ability to trust God when we cannot change or fix a situation; Ability to trust when we cannot understand what God is doing.	Well-being, sense of value, wholeness; We believe we belong to God; Believing God no matter what.
Salvation	Access to God; Free and renewed mind; Sound mind; Know the mind of Christ.	Love from the Father; Imperfections covered; Feeling loved and protected; Wholeness guaranteed; Controlled stress; Not confused.
Word of God	To know God's authority, His commands, provision, and promises; Offensive and defensive weapon; Ability to execute the power and promises of Christ in our life.	Expectation, assurance, and confidence; Disease-free, strong frame, and wisdom.
Prayer	Constant communion with God the Father.	Obedience to God's instructions; Immune response is peace that eliminates stress; Power of Jesus; Wholeness; Strength; Joy.

As we walk in love, sometimes we may appear more vulnerable to verbal attacks and abuse. Sometimes these attacks, the "fiery darts" mentioned in verse 16, come from people who are close to you like a spouse or child.

Sometimes darts hit as we go about our day. Words that are least expected can pierce, sting, and hurt your feelings.

One day, I was driving and got off the exit ramp from the freeway. I looked in my rearview mirror and behind me was a car with a man who was very angry and outraged, with the gestures to match! At the next traffic light, he stopped beside my car and yelled the most unexpected words of anger and hatred toward me. I never knew what I did to bring on such behavior. But I was glad I had the shield of faith to prevent me from absorbing those words into my spirit and mind. We walk daily with the shield of faith so that we are protected from emotional hits.

Living well is a lifestyle and a battle. Our life, however, must exist outside of the diseased culture. The Bible states that we are in the world but we are not of this world (John 17:15-16). Impossible? Is there anything impossible for God? No.

The life outside of the diseased culture is one that is built on the truth of life. We know that our Creator God, the all-powerful, eternal force, and universal intelligence, is love and truth. Many Christians have willfully jumped into the battle for being well. They have the expectation of feeling better every day, a sense of urgency of purpose, and a deep desire to understand and obey the will of God for their lives.

> The world is unprincipled. It's dog-eat-dog out there! The world doesn't fight fair. But we don't live or fight our battles that way—never have and never will. The tools of our trade aren't for marketing or manipulation, but they are for demolishing that entire massively corrupt culture. We use our powerful God-tools for smashing warped philosophies, tearing down barriers erected against the truth of God, fitting every loose thought and emotion and impulse into the structure of life shaped by Christ. Our tools are ready at hand for clearing the ground of every obstruction and building lives of obedience into maturity.
> —II Corinthians 10:3-6

 I am in a battle for wellness, but I am equipped with the best weapons.

 The battle is within every decision that I make.

THE
WELLNESS
BATTLE PLAN

"So here's what I want you to do, God helping you: Take your everyday, ordinary life—your sleeping, eating, going-to-work, and walking-around life—and place it before God as an offering. Embracing what God does for you is the best thing you can do for him. Don't become so well adjusted to your culture that you fit into it without even thinking. Instead, fix your attention on God. You'll be changed from the inside out. Readily recognize what he wants from you, and quickly respond to it. Unlike the culture around you, always dragging you down to its level of immaturity, God brings the best out of you, develops well-formed maturity in you." —Romans 12:1-2

W e have discussed the fact that wellness is a lifestyle and that life itself is a gift based on the incredible love of God. We also discussed how essential it is to embrace God's love. We understand the attributes of God are a trinity, which consists of the Father, Son, and Holy Spirit, and likewise we have been made to reflect that trinity with our mind, body, and spirit. Therefore, we are a trinity also. A reflection is not independent of its source. We have also made a commitment to Jesus the Christ, who has repaired our broken relationship with God the Father.

We cannot, then, be complete without the ongoing connection to God. Our very nature has been wired to God by God. And when the connection was broken, God fused it back together permanently and perfectly through His son Jesus Christ. This makes us children of God. This fix is available to anyone who chooses to be well. It is the truth, and it is common sense about wellness.

The cure to sickness, disease, and all kinds of trouble is older than anyone reading this book. Think about it: what kind of creator would create something, then watch it fall apart with no thought as to how it should be held together? Children of God should be the healthiest people on the face of the Earth. Others should point to them with a desire to be well. But we know that there are few opportunities for others to see Christians walking in wellness. We can change this and become that "salt of the earth," the beacons of light who draw all of humanity to the One who gives us wellness. So we can conclude if God is in all of life, He has a good understanding of what wellness is all about. We need to understand this path.

From a strategic point of view, our health is far more important than our retirement portfolio. Wealth without wellness means that someone else will enjoy your wealth after you die of a disease. If you were to envision what you would like to be doing and how you would want to be living 10 or 20 years from now, what would that be? In order to get there, we must envision the path and the plan that will help us achieve that goal. With God's help, our vision and path will become clearer. We can pursue it with a sense of urgency and excitement!

Framework for Living

> His love has taken over our lives; God's faithful ways are eternal. Thank God because He's good, because His love never quits.
> —Psalms 117:2; 118:1

Authentic wellness can be summed up in three basic wellness principles:

1. **Wellness is a common-sense lifestyle.**

   Wellness engages our minds, bodies, and spirits to live and embrace truth. These truths are more than just the facts that "birds fly" and "bees sting." It is the truth about God and all of His creation. There is a natural, inherent tendency for higher-functioning beings (humans) to maintain stability and avoid any situation or stimulus that would disturb normal functioning. The diseased culture has severely disturbed our normal functioning, preventing us from achieving wellness and knowing the truth (God). But when we strip away that diseased culture and our own confusion, we know that wellness is a common-sense lifestyle, and we know instinctively that wellness is found through a higher power that is God the Father. Through God, we can reconnect with the truth that leads us to wellness.

2. **Wellness is built upon love within the Kingdom of God.**

    When Jesus' love built the bridge leading us back to the Father, he brought the Kingdom of God to earth for us to dwell therein. This Kingdom is one that the eyes cannot see, however it stretches wide and encompasses all who believe in Jesus. Its borders are secure. The Word of God establishes the rules and lifestyle of its inhabitants. The atmosphere and energy source of the Kingdom is the power of God, and in it, we move and have our being. Children of God are captured by the diseased culture when they attempt life outside of the Kingdom.

3. **Wellness is a lifelong battle.**

    Children of God are soldiers in foreign territory. Scripture says that we are in the world but not of this world (John 17:15-16). This means that we are in the Kingdom but may work with people who are not. Our children attend school with other children who are not yet within God's Kingdom. It means that the Kingdom does not govern leadership of various institutions, including the media, grocery stores, and hospitals. Our mission to bring the light of the Kingdom to a falsely lit world causes continuous conflict. Children of God who are not mindful of this are vulnerable because the enemy of God never loses track of God's children.

> Every word of God proves true. He is a shield to all who come to Him for protection. —Proverbs 30:5 (NLT)

These principles are foundational for building the mind's habit for conscious living and the pursuit of wellness. We can build upon these principles as we transition and develop our personal battle plan.

Many things impact wellness, such as what we think, what we do, our genetic code, and the environment. We must begin by implementing small but permanent changes that gradually move us into a state of wellness. I have found that drastic swings of change do not work over time because they often lack the foundation that is required for permanent change. As we sharpen the gift of common sense, with clear thinking and logical action regarding our current state, we will get stronger and be able to react faster when making corrections to maintain personal wellness.

God provides the framework for successful living. So how do we live and keep our trinity—our reflection of God—well in the midst of a vicious war? God has provided the protections, instructions, agreements, benefits, insurances, examples, and guarantees for life. All of the details for wellness are outlined in the Word of God, the Holy Bible. According to John 1:1-14, "Jesus—the Word, the Intelligence, the Grace, and the Christ—was in the beginning and the Word became flesh." Remember that the Trinity of God from the beginning included the attributes of the Christ. As we pursue this answer, we will look at each attribute of our trinity. We need to know the vulnerable points of each attribute and what weapons are available to us to protect them. We then will apply the Seven Disciplines of Wellness that bring these attributes into the framework with application for us to live and sustain our wellness. The wellness battle plan is a powerful tool to help us develop the right habits, drive alignment to our purpose (God's will for us), and put accountability into the way we live each day.

The Mind – The Battlefield

A healthy mind is one that thinks. The mind is not a receptacle or dumping ground for whatever the enemy chooses to deposit. A healthy mind avoids certain exposures and synthesizes information for truth and the will of God. It prayerfully processes stress and violations, practices seeing the good in situations and people, and uses Scripture and healthy relationships to stay well.

> Let this mind be in you which was also in Christ Jesus.
> —Philippians 2:5 (KJV)

The battlefield for wellness is within our minds. The mind is where choice, intelligence, vision, thought, decision, and feeling impact our trinity. The state of the body reflects behaviors based on thought, choice, and instinct. One of the key weapons for battle is the helmet of salvation (Ephesians 6:17), which is the protector of the head and in this instance, relates to the mind and the protection we have because of the saving gift of Christ. This means that you do not ever have to lose your mind, nor can your mind be taken from you! There are some important precautionary measures we should take to reduce our vulnerability to the attacks against our minds by the enemy. The most important measure is having knowledge of the Word of God concerning your mental health. A healthy mind makes choices and decisions that are in line with the will and purposes of God.

Vulnerable Point: Leadership

The enemy, in his efforts to keep us disconnected from God, presents new leadership and other inferior gods. Once these are in place, it is easy for us to fill the yearning of our soul for God with these gods. Charles Allen states in his book *God's Psychiatry*, "Man is incomplete without an object to worship. The flow of a river cannot be stopped, however the channel in which it flows can be diverted." We divert our worship toward other gods. Allen continues, "There are five objects of worship which multitudes today have put before God: wealth, fame, pleasure, power, and knowledge." Allen points out that our worship of wealth never makes us satisfied. Fame causes us to go to extremes to get attention. Pleasure is addictive and thought to be the key to happiness. Worship of personal power ends up hurting people. Worshiping knowledge leads to disobedience against God.

Counter Attack: Warrior Mind-set

One of the first rules for life given to Moses by God for the Israelite people was "You shall have no other gods before me" (Exodus 20:3, NIV). We are wired at creation to worship God. He is a very jealous God and will not compete for His rightful place (Exodus 20:5). To be well is to have the right leadership in our lives. Knowing God helps us know who we are. Knowing "who we are in Christ" gives us the power to change. God is our

Creator, Father, Savior, and Friend. God has the intelligence needed to survive enemy territory. He knows where all the land mines of life are buried. The right leadership provides reinforcement and a protective presence during battle and in times of peace.

Vulnerable Point: Negative Thought

Negativity drains our energy. It is also habit-forming. Negative thought is a very natural part of diseased culture thinking. This behavior is a virus permitted to spread from top to bottom in our society. The glass being half-empty is confirmed everywhere we go. Nothing good is acceptable, including us. Self-hate is a major asset in the diseased culture. Negative thinking is not characteristic of a healthy mind. Thoughts are so powerful that once conceived, they can quickly become a reality. Thoughts take us places; where our thoughts go, our emotions follow.

Dr. Catherine Ponder says, "Every word brings forth after its kind; first in mind, then in body, and later in the affairs of the individual." In his book *You Can't Afford the Luxury of a Negative Thought*, Pete McWilliams writes, "Thoughts have power over our mind, our body, and our emotions. Positive thoughts (joy, happiness, fulfillment, achievement, worthiness) have positive results (enthusiasm, calm, well-being, ease, energy, love). Negative thoughts (judgment, unworthiness, mistrust, resentment, fear) produce negative results (tension, anxiety, alienation, anger, fatigue)."

Counter Attack: Warrior Mind-set

One sure way to combat negative thinking is to practice the "grateful heart" technique. The grateful heart technique identifies those things we have to be appreciative of and thankful for. With this, we can walk in obedience to God's Word, which says "In everything give thanks: for this is the will of God in Christ Jesus concerning you" (1 Thessalonians 5:18 KJV). We also know that things could be worse. The apostle and pastor Paul in Scripture admonishes us in Philippians 4:8:

> "Friends, I'd say you'll do best by filling your minds and meditating on things true, noble, reputable, authentic, compelling, gracious—the

best, not the worst; the beautiful, not the ugly; things to praise, not things to curse."

We need to focus on putting positive things in our minds instead of negative ones.

A thought is like a coin; it has a head (positive) and a tail (negative).

Vulnerable Point: Imagination

One essential element of the thought process is the work of the imagination. The partner to negative thinking is misuse of imagination. The imagination is one of the most powerful attributes of the mind. It was designed by God to stimulate a series of thoughts and conclusions, feeding our values and leading to good behaviors. The brain collects millions of images in our lifetime. All of these images impact us in some manner. We are constantly being presented with images of fear, poverty, disease, and pornography. This is the danger of television, movies, and the Internet: they can be anti-wellness. They shape our minds and thoughts and influence our values.

When we are constantly presented with these unrealistic images, it is easy to remain in survival mode, the low-brain point where thought is minimal. Life and how we experience it, then, is based on the images already stored in the brain. We retrieve them and apply them to our situation, be it the lifestyle of the rich and famous, high fashion, or the latest doll or action hero. The image could be weight loss by not eating carbs or being a desperate (lustful) housewife. The enemy also distorts the use of our imaginations by our desire to have gods that we can see, including technology, houses, relationships, cars, or fraternities. They become gods when they are selfishly placed before God the Father—all driven by the enemy's influence on our imaginations.

Seek ye first the Kingdom of God, and His righteousness; and all these things shall be added unto you. —Matthew 6:33 (KJV)

Counter Attack: Warrior Mind-set

In order to be well, it is very important to guard our imaginations against constant exposure to images that do not agree with our wellness way of living. It makes it easy to compare ourselves to others and develop a false standard of perfection that cannot be met. The image we have of ourselves is vulnerable to our imagination and those images we entertain. These images affect our ability to love and appreciate ourselves. It is not a good idea to allow Hollywood or Wall Street to have that much influence on our ability to live well. God commands: "You must not make for yourself an idol of any kind or an image of anything in the heavens or on the earth or in the sea" (Deuteronomy 5:8, NLT). Therefore, we must fit every loose thought, emotion, and impulse into the structure of life shaped by God and His Word.

As we learn about the life of Jesus, we can see ourselves well, thriving with purpose, rooted in love and uninhibited about the possibilities for greatness that each day brings. I have come to realize that no two days are alike with Christ. We need to receive each day as the gift that it is. Everywhere we look, we can see God. The sun rises differently every day. It changes the colors of the sky, the largest piece of canvas ever known. The sunset is beyond description and is the perfect ending to a day filled with opportunities, in which we flow with whatever the Creator presented— opportunities for us to react, remaining confident in love and in the wellness habits that we fine-tune every day.

> Casting down imaginations, and every high thing that exalteth itself against the knowledge of God, and bringing into captivity every thought to the obedience of Christ. —II Corinthians 10:5 (KJV)

Vulnerable Point: Low-Brain Thinking

In the absence of thought, humans become animalistic, living primarily upon instinct. At birth, animals possess instinctive behaviors. An instinct is a response to a stimulus that is inborn; no training is needed. Instinct is what animals use to survive. Hunger or the threat of a natural predator will automatically trigger a timely response, but not at the conscious level. In mating, some animals are adorned with distinctive colors and scents within their species that attract the opposite sex. Their babies are born to know how to nurse. And so it is with humans.

Humans, however, are quite different in their cognitive makeup than other animals. In addition to instinct, we can think and make choices. We build societies, groups of people who live in an organized fashion. In the absence of core values and a belief system rooted in love, our lower brain (instincts) can be overstimulated, causing us to act out instinctive behaviors. Earl Nightingale, in his famous recording "The Strangest Secret," states that "you become what you think about." As a result, the consequences for those behaviors play out. People go to jail, others get divorced, children are hurt, careers are ruined, and people become discouraged. How many times have you heard someone ask, "What was he thinking?" The answer: he was not thinking!

Big business has mastered the ability to appeal to our instincts, overriding thought and training us to ignore common sense. That way, we can be herded into behaviors that are most profitable for them.

The desire to eat can be triggered by food photography or commercials, even if the viewer is not hungry. The threat of catastrophes (i.e. terrorist attack, natural disaster) or giving into fear-mongering (i.e. sensationalist news reporting) induce higher stress levels and raise blood pressure. The fear of being alone justifies toxic relationships. When the instinct to procreate is stimulated, many people become caught up in the realm of pornography and sexual promiscuity. In the absence of higher brain function, like thought and self-control, the mindless response to daily experiences shape our behaviors, habits, and mental capacity to stay well. Our reaction to fear keeps us at the low-brain point, which provides very little cognitive abilities. As a result, destructive behavior is oftentimes the response. Acting out of instinct conditions us to behave based on the agendas of others.

Counter Attack: Warrior Mind-set

A person without **self-control** is like a house with its doors and windows knocked out. —Proverbs 25:28

Humans have the capacity to relate to internal experiences like thoughts, as well as external experiences like sunsets. We are the reflection of God.

We can identify inner feelings and relate them to others. We can connect those feelings to the past, present, and future. We have the ability to execute complex sequences of behavior needed for employment and building societies. As a result, we can have expectations and make choices. When decisions are made, they are logical, high-brain thinking is clear, and memory function is stronger. We can use self-control and delay gratification by weighing consequences. We can also choose to limit our exposure to the things that perpetuate dysfunctions.

Vulnerable Point: Living at Capacity

The challenge with our existing way of living is that we have the ability to get more done much faster, so we can take more on. With the many tools of technology, we have developed a false sense of being able to handle it all. We rarely see the need to say, "No, that is enough!" It is a strategy of the enemy for us to remain busy, overcommitted, and chronically stressed. We constantly exceed the limits of our trinity. Our ability to survive the unexpected is threatened. There is little room for staying well.

Counter Attack: Warrior Mind-set

> And be not conformed to this world: but be ye transformed by the renewing of your mind. —Romans 12:2 (KJV)

In order to be well and stay well over the years, we must have the **capacity** to do so. This means that within the mind, body, and spirit, there should be reserves that permit us to deal with life's hills and valleys without tipping the scale toward a health challenge. In a diseased culture, living at full capacity appears to be an unconscious but normal way of living. This was not God's intent and we were not designed for such behavior.

> Jesus gives us the ultimate rest, the confidence we need, to escape the frustration and chaos of the world around us. —Billy Graham

Vulnerable Point: Resistant to Change

Change can be stressful. It can be positive, but in many cases, it is viewed as something negative. Most change is difficult and unpredictable. It is uncomfortable for most of us and we would rather live without it. Change can be frightening, even good change. It threatens the familiar and breaks our habits. If the enemy can make us resistant to change, we become more rigid in our bad thinking and we become trapped inside bad habits such as eating poorly, smoking, staying in toxic relationships, abusing alcohol, and so on. We fear what life would be like without these familiar yet unhealthy habits. The fear and negative self-talk about the unknown is what locks us in. We think that it is better to be miserable than to be with the unknown. The clincher: spending time with the miserable to reinforce our status quo behaviors.

Growing older is another weapon of change used against us on the wellness path. Anyone who has negative feelings about getting older is in trouble. Trying to stay young may be the primary root cause of our health challenges. When we attempt to be something that we are not, the landscape of truth is altered as well as the love within us.

> "For I know the plans I have for you," says the Lord. "They are plans for good and not for disaster, to give you a future and a hope."
> —Jeremiah 29:11 (NLT)

Counter Attack: Warrior Mind-set

Our most important change is embracing God's everlasting love for us and His plan for our lives. Change is inevitable and necessary, but it's also exciting! It brings good times as well as hard times.

The changing of the seasons provides a mental health exercise for letting go of what was and adapting to the new. Summer can try to hang around, but autumn will not allow it to keep center stage; it pushes summer out of the way! We cannot hold on to the past. Seasons remind us that God is in charge. Change brings hope to our future.

We must have faith to embrace change. Change can signal a new beginning: a fresh start and an opportunity to do things better the second time around. It requires trust in God to remember that things will work for your greater good. Change is timely, like the seasons.

> I love God and He loves me. His purpose is my purpose. I am safe and at peace with change. A healthy spirit supports my mental capacity to handle change. —S.A.J.

Vulnerable Point: Misunderstanding Mental Health

The World Health Organization defines mental health as not just the absence of a mental disorder, but as a state of well-being in which every individual realizes his or her own potential, can cope with the normal stresses of life, can work productively and fruitfully, and is able to make a contribution to his or her community.

This definition implies that there is a foundation that provides the capacity to think, make good decisions, and move through the ups and downs of life. We need the ability to reason, manage, and build on our day-to-day experiences.

Mental disorders are prevalent in the United States. According to the National Institute of Mental Health, an estimated 26.2 percent of Americans ages 18 and older suffer from a diagnosable mental disorder in a given year. This means that approximately 57.7 million people ages 18 and older have a mental disorder. In addition, mental disorders are the number one cause of disability in the U.S. and Canada for ages 15-44.

In a diseased culture, more time is spent discussing mental illness as opposed to mental health. As a result, we have fragments of treatments and bandages for dealing with those things that threaten our mental health.

Mental health can be impacted in ways similar to our physical health. When we break a leg, the whole body goes into trauma. We get X-rays to determine the extent of the break. We reduce the blood flow and swelling with compresses to decrease pain. We then secure the leg for healing and protection against re-injury. If we have an experience where someone was intentionally abusive, this emotional injury affects our mental health. The mind will attempt to restore itself. Emotional injuries can raise blood pressure and cause tears, perspiration, muscle tension, shakes, insomnia, edginess, and irritation. These symptoms can last for a few days or longer as the mind processes the trauma and begins to heal.

There is a stigma attached to someone who experiences a mental disorder. The risk factors for poor mental health include chronic stress, mental overload, unresolved issues, toxic relationships, poor eating habits, and substance abuse. They can become the catalyst for the physical presentation of disease over time. These conditions are rarely seen as the root cause of the physical ailment.

Counter Attack: Warrior Mind-set

> And be **renewed** in the spirit of your mind.
> —Ephesians 4:23 (KJV)

Seeking additional help from pastoral counselors, therapists, and Christian support groups are all options to restore mental health. Getting treatment helps speed up the recovery time by providing an objective view of your situation. It can also help pinpoint unresolved issues of the past that could be the root cause to the ailment. Prayer for guidance and protection is essential as you seek treatment.

A healthy diet is also important for supporting mental health and recovery. Chemical imbalances can be caused by the lack of nutrients.

Summary: The Mind Is the Battlefield

Until we learn to care for our entire trinity, we cannot be complete and well. We can eat as many fruits and vegetables as humanly possible. We can work out at the gym faithfully. Or we can use the best supplements and pharmaceuticals, creating the illusion of good health and well-being. With all this, we have the perfect book cover. But we are solely treating the body and neglecting the inside. As we expose our minds to truth and love, the path to wellness will become conscious and clear without confusion.

Tools for Maintaining Mental Health

Know your value system	Based on your belief in God and His love and Word. Replay and nourish it with like-minded people. Compare your values against those of the diseased culture.
Healthy images	Observe all of nature—all that God created. "Yet I am confident I will see the Lord's goodness while I am here in the land of the living." (Ps. 27:13, NLT)
Time management	Manage capacity. If you are too busy to maintain your connection to God, then you are too busy to remain well or live. "To every thing there is a season, and a time to every purpose under the heaven." (Eccl. 3:1, KJV)
Staying in the moment	"Do not worry about tomorrow, for tomorrow will bring issues of its own." (Matt. 6:34)
Thoughts	Thoughts are a choice, and we can change the script. Pray about your imagination and anything you don't have the answers to. Using Scripture several times each day will help restore our thought life. What to think on is outlined in Philippians 4:8.
Internal conversations	What we say to ourselves can hurt and reinforce negative, life-draining ideas. Opt to say the encouraging, loving things that bring energy and hope.
Fear	"For God hath not given us the spirit of fear; but of power, and of love, and of a sound mind." (II Tim. 1:7, KJV) "The name of the LORD is a strong tower: the righteous runneth into it, and is safe." (Prov. 18:10, KJV)
Releasing the need to worry	"Casting all your care upon him; for he careth for you" (1 Pet. 5:7, KJV). We pray about concerns. Worry demonstrates a lack of faith.
Truth about feelings	Honesty, when practiced, will get easier. We will see that honesty to God the Father about our feelings is encouraged. He knows what is on our hearts and in our minds anyway. "The truth shall make you free." (John 8:32, KJV).
Healthy relationships	"A man that hath friends must show himself friendly: and there is a friend that sticketh closer than a brother." (Prov. 18:24, KJV) "You use steel to sharpen steel, and one friend sharpens another." (Prov. 27:17)
Forgiveness	Hard to do but possible through Christ. We must forgive others and ourselves. We must also realize that we need to forgive in order to be forgiven. "For if ye forgive men their trespasses, your heavenly Father will also forgive you." (Matt. 6:14, KJV)
Embracing change	All change is not good. Yet change is inevitable. Seek the will of God to assist you during times of change.

Body Battles

Christian author Richard Foster once said, "Our body is a portable sanctuary through which we are daily experiencing the presence of God." Our body, according to Psalm 139:15-16, is the outer shell for the trinity of man, designed by God.

> "You know me inside and out, you know every bone in my body; you
> know exactly how I was made, bit by bit, how I was sculpted from
> nothing into something."

"The body is not the person, but rather the external case that houses the person," say Drs. Chester Tolson and Harold Koenig in their book *The Healing Power of Prayer*. The body is the physical representation of the reflection of God. It parallels the Holy Spirit of God, "the doer or executor" of God's will. We are tools in the hand of God designed to carry out the work we were created to do.

Don't you realize that your body is the temple of the Holy Spirit, who lives in you and was given to you by God? You do not belong to yourself.
—I Corinthians 6:19 (NLT)

The body is made up of many cells. While no exact number can be agreed upon, it is estimated that the adult human body contains 75 to 100 trillion cells. And "bit by bit," God watched over us as we were being formed in the wombs of our mothers (Psalm 139:13-16). Individually, each cell and its makeup reflect the function of the whole body. Each cell absorbs nutrients and throws off waste. Cells have intelligence and memory. They speak, listen, move, and follow instructions. Cells also contain the genetic inscription that makes each of us unique.

The body is also self-healing. A healthy body is one that takes the good you feed it—be it spiritual, mental, or physical—and heals itself. It is constantly monitoring itself with a built-in immune system to protect and correct any malfunction. The body is designed to respond to threats against any member of our trinity. Spirit or mind, the body is involved. It is handcrafted to monitor and protect the health and well-being of the whole person. For example, WebMD and the Mayo Clinic list chronic stress and inactivity as two of the risk factors for high blood pressure. Stress relates to how we process things mentally, but it also changes levels of the body's hormones, including adrenaline, cortisone, and cortisol. Studies also link stress to changes in blood sugar levels and immune function. Inactivity relates to the lack of physical conditioning of the body and as a result, the heart rate increases and works harder to send blood through the arteries. Same diagnosis—high blood pressure from two different origins—one physical, one mental. When the trinity of a person is threatened, the body will carry the message and the response.

> When God lives and breathes in you (and He does, as surely as He did in Jesus), you are delivered from that dead life. With His Spirit living in you, your body will be as alive as Christ's! —Romans 8:11

Vulnerable Point: Chronic Stressors

I have discovered many people do not feel that they are under a lot of stress and they reject the fact that stress could be the root cause of the physical problem they are experiencing. It is difficult to manage something if we do not know what it is. So what is stress?

Stress is the body's response to change, be it good or bad. Change is constant. It could be stress on your daughter's wedding day, receiving that job promotion, or the birth of your baby. It could be the worst of divorces or a child in rebellion. Not all stress is bad. We need stress when danger is present. It triggers the body's ability to react quickly by supplying the hormones, elevated blood pressure, and energy that is needed to escape. This is referred to as the **fight-or-flight** response. We all have different stressors. For example, you may find jumping out of airplanes to be one of the most exciting things in life. On the other hand, I find the thought horrifying. I can take roadway abuse without becoming a "road rager" myself. For someone else, being disrespected by another driver could be the last straw. Short-term stress is considered normal and necessary for survival, and we all have different triggers and different ways of handling it.

The type of stress that we must avoid and manage is **chronic stress**. This is when the fight-or-flight response is activated so often that the body doesn't always have a chance to return to normal. It can be like a fire hose adding pressure to circumstances and situations, many of which are beyond our control but constant. The biggest stressors include lack of resources, time, money, toxic relationships, poor health, loneliness, change, and guilt. Chronic stress is poison. The **physical signs** could be general aches and pains, grinding teeth, or clenched jaws. We may experience headaches, indigestion, difficulty sleeping, racing heart, ringing in the ears, sweaty palms, poor posture, or upset stomach. There are also certain behaviors associated with stress that may include being critical of others, relationship hopping, impulsive actions, eating disorders, argumentativeness, road rage, or substance abuse. Emotional and mental indicators include lack of concentration, worry, fear, anger, anxiety, and memory loss. Depression, seclusion, and negative attitudes can also be signs of chronic stress. The **spiritual signs** of stress include hopelessness, loneliness, negative thoughts, low self-esteem, and fear.

We learned earlier that the body represents the response of the whole person and will therefore display the mind and spirit's response to stress. Chronic stress is a major risk factor for many physical and mental complications, and is something we all experience at some point in our lives.

Counter Attack: Warrior Mind-set

> Let this mind be in you, which was also in Christ Jesus.
> —Philippians 2:5 (KJV)

Managing stress requires personal intervention using some very basic thoughts and a prayer life to help put things in perspective. A key thought: if God is aware of all that is going on, why should I get so worked up about it? He allowed it, and I trust Him! **Stress is a poison. Prayer manages stress.**

Vulnerable Point: Malnutrition

Malnutrition doesn't just mean lack of food. Malnutrition is the lack of micronutrients, including a range of vitamins, minerals, and good fat. As a result, eating large amounts of foods that lack these nutrients leads to obesity. When these nutrients are not available, our brain and nervous system are negatively impacted.

The brain is very much affected by what we eat. If we skip meals, eat lots of sugar and red meat, or drink caffeine with little water, we weaken the brain and the entire nervous system. Too much sugar negatively impacts blood sugar levels and our ability to think and reason. Dysfunctional blood sugar and hormone levels also negatively influence our mental capacity and our ability to feel strong and at peace.

Counter Attack: Warrior Mind-set

There is a relationship between what we eat and how we feel and think. We choose to eat to live and live well in order to stay strong, make good decisions, and glorify God the Father. When we eat good proteins like fish, whole grains, raw fruits and vegetables, nuts and beans, and drink plenty of water, we have provided the brain what it needs to function well.

Vulnerable Point: Destructive Habits

A part of the enemy's strategy is to get us to develop destructive thoughts and habits, such as poor eating, overeating, not sleeping, drugs, and wild living. Over time, these habits force the body to self-destruct through some type of sickness or disease. The more chronic the disease and the longer and more pronounced the disease, the more wear and tear it will have on a person, his or her family, and caregivers. For the enemy, the goal in battle is that soldiers, at worst, are wounded, not killed. A wounded soldier requires the attention of other soldiers (at least two) to carry the wounded one off to safety. Just with one hit, at least three soldiers are disabled, distraught, discouraged, or traumatized. This scenario can be devastating to one's family, friends, and coworkers. Even though the body is self-healing, modern medicine has become the standard approach to everything. Natural medicine, which encourages and supports the self-healing nature of the body, is seen as quackery in some circles. Chronic diseases are the perfect weapons; their effect is far-reaching and is being sustained by key economic components of the diseased culture.

Sexual Promiscuity

Another destructive habit is sexual promiscuity. In Scripture, it is a violation, not just against God, but against our own body. We know that the cost of sin is death, which is why we need Christ (Romans 6:23). We fail to consider that sex by design engages the whole trinity. Many of us violate our bodies with sexual sins with deep consequences that devalue and bring out animalistic, low-brain behavior. Sex outside of marriage is trespassing against a sacred vessel. This collision causes emotional injury and distorts that reflection of God in our spirit and the body, though our emotions carry the weight.

Poor Use of Time: Too Busy

Time is a resource that most of us lack. We are so busy. We react to things instead of planning for them. We are fully committed to the agenda of others and not one consciously developed for our family and ourselves. The busier we are, the better we feel. Whenever there is an open slot of time, it must be filled immediately! While some of us see this type of behavior as a symbol of success, I see it as an unconscious addiction to chaos. Many of us fear silence, being alone, and having few demands or crises, but if we remain busy, there is no time to plan, reflect, change, deal with past hurts, or think deeply about those things that move us forward in life.

Based on what we know about our loving God, the lack-of-time issue resembles some other strategies of the enemy. It is another drain on our ability to be well. Some of the damaging takeaways include chronic diseases and no time to pray, eat properly, sleep, or spend with family.

Poor Use of Time: Too Bored

Boredom can be another serious time waster. Boredom is an emotional state where a person lacks focus, motivation, or interest in his or her current surroundings. This fits nicely in a world where negativity and disappointment are all around. Television and other mindless pursuits of arousal are used to pass the time. This often leads to sexual promiscuity, substance abuse, and overeating, which all weaken the body.

Eating Too Much or Too Little

The habit of eating too much high-calorie, high-fat, and highly refined carbohydrate food and too little of fresh fruits, vegetables, and whole grains is far too convenient. Poor food choices are all around. If we stop for gasoline on a trip, there are soda and chips to fill the gap until dinner. There is too much cheap, tasty, poor quality food and too little of the nutrient-rich food we need.

Food as a Multiuse Item

Today, food in many instances is a multiuse item. Food is the friend that won't talk back or criticize; it is the reward after a long struggle or hard day at work. Food is used as the draw to increase attendance at events. Eating goes way beyond hunger or the need for nourishment.

Lack of Exercise

A consistent exercise routine is very hard to maintain when there is a poor diet, which lowers energy levels and causes weight gain. Chronic stress can change the hormone levels which reinforces overweight conditions. Sleep deprivation can cause low energy that leads to painful, sometimes inflamed joints—all of which discourage exercise. What a trap!

> God rescued us from dead-end alleys and dark dungeons. He's set us up in the Kingdom of the Son. He loves so much, the Son who got us out of the pit we were in, got rid of the sins we were doomed to keep repeating.
> —Colossians 1:13-14

Counter Attack: Warrior Mind-set

Some people think that they can basically live carefree and that whatever breaks, modern medicine and technology will be able to fix it! Most problems cannot be fixed. Many of them can be patched up, but with drastic reductions in quality and length of life. It is not God's will for us to be sick. Jesus used much of his time healing and caring for the sick and diseased. He understood that trinity health was key to glorifying the Father with our lives. As he healed, Jesus would speak life to whatever attribute of the trinity was diseased. He would say to the sick in spirit, "Go and sin no more" (John 8:11, KJV). To the sick in mind, "Thy faith hath made thee whole" (Matthew 9:22, KJV), and to the sick in body, "Take up thy bed and walk" (Mark 2:9, KJV). Know that Jesus stood in our place on the cross to cover all sin, sickness, and disease. His shed blood for us restores health to all who embrace him.

> The body is the report card of how we have used the gift of life.
> —S.A.J.

Prayer for the Body

"Lord, forgive me for mistreating the wonderful body you gave to me. A body to love, care for, and complete the special work you have for me. Help me to make the changes I need to regain my health and be a good example for my family. Body, mind, and spirit, I yield completely. I can't do this without your help. I will follow your lead. I will give you the praise in Jesus' name. Amen."

Spirit Battle

> There is no room in love for fear. Well-formed love banishes fear. Since fear is crippling, a fearful life—fear of death, fear of judgment—is one not yet fully formed in love. —I John 4:18

In order to win the battle for wellness, we must spend time with the Lord and study our orders in the Bible. "The Bible is spiritual food, which must be metabolized in order to live a spiritual life," says Larry Wood. A healthy spirit recognizes that it is not God and that God is greater. The evidence of our relationship with the Father is that we reflect the attributes of the Holy Spirit within us. The evidence, or fruit, of the spirit includes greater love, peace, joy, patience, gentleness, goodness, meekness, temperance, and faith (Galatians 5:22-23). A healthy spirit acknowledges God every day with gratitude and seeks to please Him.

Some of us acknowledge God by damning Him or by telling God to damn others; that is not healthy. A healthy spirit realizes its vulnerability and is grateful for all that it cannot do for itself. A healthy spirit helps develop a healthy mind, which, in turn, supports a healthy body.

A healthy spirit can look at nature and see the wonder of God! Like the leaves on the trees in autumn and the painted clouds of a sunset, we too have colors. Our "true colors" shape our value systems. Through our value systems, we live vibrantly and full of energy, or we go through the motions of life, dull and lackluster. Our spirits reflect our true colors, which show through in how we treat our Creator, ourselves, each other, and the Earth.

> With his stripes, we are healed. —Isaiah 53:5 (KJV)

Vulnerable Point: Weak in Spirit

Hard times and challenges have a way of taking our attention away from the Father and embracing the fear and problem-solving norms within the diseased culture. When we doubt our relationship and confidence in our position with the Father, we lose the potential for staying well. We lose the ability to be productive and to know peace. Our witness is weaker, our zeal for life on God's terms fades, and therefore we are neutralized.

The enemy's most successful weapon to the natural order of life as God designed it is rebellion and disobedience, which produces discouragement and hopelessness. He uses our desire for perfection to lead us into situations and things that set us up for disappointment. When we fall or make mistakes, we must run to God and not run from Him.

It is also critical to the enemy that we devalue ourselves and forget who and whose we are, thus mistreating ourselves. We look for love in all the wrong places and settle for less.

Counter Attack: Warrior Mind-set

> There is no room in love for fear. Well-formed love banishes fear. Since fear is crippling, a fearful life—fear of death, fear of judgment—is one not yet fully formed in love. —I John 4:18

Life is a privilege and a perfect gift from God. Life without this realization is like constantly driving your car in reverse. In reverse, we are physical creatures looking for answers and a possible spiritual experience of sorts. God's love would have us realize that we are spiritual creatures living a short physical existence for His glory, filled with love and purpose for the greater good. We must also remember that He is the owner of spirit, mind, and body.

The health of our spirit after accepting Christ as our Savior is perfectly aligned to God the Father. As we move toward him, he restores us *holistically*. As our relationship with him develops, we are regularly reconciled to God through prayer to remain well.

Vulnerable Point: Unforgivingness (Anger)

Many of us harbor things that have been done to us. We say, "I will never forget!" Replaying them in our minds keeps them vivid and painful. Sometimes we don't remember the details; we just remember that there is something we are never going to forgive. Unforgivingness also breeds anger, and if left to fester, it worsens with time. Not forgiving also affects the mind and the body. With time, anger changes the chemical makeup and messages from the brain.

> For if ye forgive men their trespasses, your heavenly Father will also forgive you: but if ye forgive not men their trespasses, neither will your Father forgive your trespasses. —Matthew 6:14-15 (KJV)

Counter Attack: Warrior Mind-set

If we think about what the Father orchestrated in the life, death, and resurrection of Jesus, it was all about forgiveness and restoration! If God could go through all He did to bring forth forgiveness for me, I believe that He can help me forgive.

The Seven Disciplines of Wellness

> Just because something is technically legal doesn't mean that it's spiritually appropriate. If I went around doing whatever I thought I could get by with, I'd be a slave to my whims. —I Corinthians 6:12

We have become aware of the effect being in a diseased culture has on our ability to be healthy and to be in right relationship with the Father through Jesus Christ. How do we use this new awareness to get well and not give in to life as defined by the diseased culture? Now that we have a relationship with Christ, we must put our intelligence and choice back in God's hands to bring forth the plan for restoring our health and making it a plan that is enjoyable, doable, and unique for each of us. This takes discipline.

Why do we need the Seven Disciplines, and why are they disciplines rather than habits? A discipline may or may not be a habit. Habits are repetitive acts not necessarily done to provide mental or moral improvement. A discipline goes to the next level and involves self-control, sacrifice, and a specific set of behaviors that bring an expected end. Discipline also builds in a level of accountability. It is a systematic method to obtain obedience. Success on God's terms is based on knowing and obeying the knowledge of His truth. The Seven Disciplines encourage us to walk in that truth.

We need disciplines because we are in a war. The enemy's strategy is to have us make decisions against the will of God. We need a strategy to help us stay out of trouble with God and stay well. Freedom outside of God's will brings destruction. Just because you can does not mean that you should do. God gives us a framework and appoints us stewards. We need disciplines to stay within that framework in order to be well, safe, healthy, joyful, and peaceful.

As children of God, we stay well by obeying God and His Word. Ecclesiastes 12:13 states: "The last and final word is this: fear God. Do what He tells you." We need discipline to do God's will and study His Word. We need discipline to use common sense and think and live outside of the diseased culture. We need discipline to stay focused and remain on purpose. We need discipline to eat, sleep, and move properly. We also need discipline to love as commanded and to share it appropriately. One of the initial challenges I have with many of my clients is that most of what I recommend to them are common-sense activities with little to no monetary costs. Some of the activities are so simple that my clients don't believe it can make a difference.

For example, Betty, who suffered from chronic constipation, eliminated her problem by improving her posture, drinking more water, and eating two apples a day. To address her problem, Betty could have used laxatives, which forces the bowel to move and draws water out of the body.

However, re-hydration from drinking water and the internal scrubbing that takes place from the skin of the apple were much more beneficial and naturally corrective. **What the body needed 100 years ago to be healthy is what the body needs today.** We must not let the crutches of the diseased culture make us feel incapable of or excuse us from being responsible for our primary care and well-being.

Periodic illness has its uses; it can be a warning signal. The body sends pain messages and symptoms to prevent major illnesses. It will also shut us down or attempt to force rest when more resources are needed for restoration. These Seven Disciplines, when added to our lifestyle, will give us the next steps to correct those things that keep us unhealthy, sick, and tired. What is the profile of a well person, and how do we line up when it comes to wellness? These disciplines will help shape your wellness lifestyle and serve as your point of reference when you need to be realigned or get back on track.

Attempting to implement all Seven Disciplines at once may not be a good approach for the long-term success of your transition. However, implement as you are led. I recommend an approach that takes several months.

The Seven Disciplines of Wellness

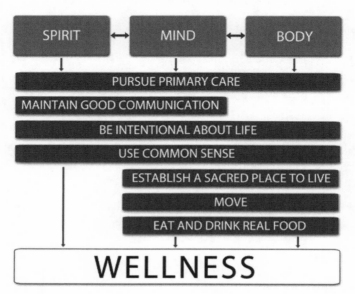

The chapters that follow provide a discussion of the disciplines and provide the interventions needed to line up to the will and way of God concerning our life within His wonderful Kingdom on Earth. In the Book of Wisdom we read, "Death is the reward of an undisciplined life; your foolish decisions trap you in a dead end" (Proverbs 5:23). From managing time to managing what we eat, the details for living well follow. Here we have the structure to walk in obedience to the plan of God. The Apostle Paul sums up the Seven Disciplines of Wellness for us in Romans 12:1-2:

> "So here's what I want you to do, God helping you: Take your everyday, ordinary life—your sleeping [**sacred place**], eating [**pure**], going-to-work, and walking-around life [**move**]—and place it before God as an offering. Embracing what God does for you is the best thing you can do for Him [**common sense**]. Don't become so well adjusted to your culture that you fit into it without even thinking. Instead, fix your attention on God [**communicate**]. You'll be changed from the inside out [**seek primary care**]. Readily recognize what he wants from you, and quickly respond to it [**be intentional**]. Unlike the culture around you, always dragging you down to its level of immaturity, God brings the best out of you, develops well-formed maturity in you [**wellness**]."

 The key to wellness is our connection to God the Father.

 I am not alone in this battle for wellness.

DISCIPLINE 1

PURSUE PRIMARY CARE

> God is love. —I John 4:8 (KJV)

A s stated previously, discipline goes beyond habit by employing self-control, sacrifice, and a specific set of behaviors that bring an expected end. Discipline also builds in a level of accountability.

So far we have concluded that God is the presence of love. We know now that God loves us and that we are His. Love is a proper noun and a verb. We need to have love as a discipline so that we can practice **loving God and consciously receiving His love. This is primary care.** We exist to reflect His love within our lives. Our living is love in action. To do anything other than love is disobedience to God, which leads to the beginning of poor health and trouble.

Primary Care Framework

> Jesus said unto him, "Thou shalt love the Lord thy God with all thy heart, and with all thy soul, and with all thy mind. This is the first and great commandment. And the second is like unto it, thou shalt love thy neighbor as thyself." —Matthew 22:37-39 (KJV)

Jesus commanded us who seek wellness and a bountiful life to love. He provided many examples by his life. He put love in three essential categories: love God the Father, love ourselves as His children, and love others. We receive love from Him in order to love others and ourselves.

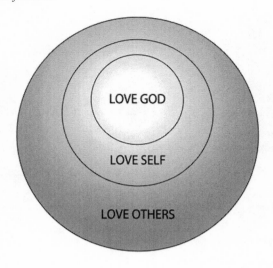

With this commandment, we have the keys to live well, on purpose, and in peace. Life can be much simpler than many of us have come to know it. We are on our way to wellness when we enter into the relationship outlined in this commandment—loving God for who He is, for what He has done, and believing that He is and that He will do all that He promises in Scripture. When we love God, He will show us how to love others and ourselves authentically.

Receiving Primary Care

God loved us even when we were not acting very lovable. His love was not based on a condition. Whether we loved Him or not, He still loved us and gave Jesus up to bring us back to Him. Now that we are aware of this love, God says, "Love me first. Let me see me in you." Our neglect and casual acknowledgment of God breaks His heart. Adam and Eve, who were first in their disobedience, broke His heart, but He loved them through it (Genesis 3:9-24). The children of Israel, the people He had set apart for Himself, were next when they asked for a king that they could see—a mere human. These precious people forgot that God gave them the eyes they used to see and the very oxygen they breathed. But He loved them through that (1 Samuel 10:17-24, 11:15). Even we, in our continual disobedience and god-like entitlement behavior, were remedied when Jesus took the penalty of our sin, demonstrating a love that is inconceivable. We can never earn God's love; it is a precious gift. Our obedience to His commands is how we demonstrate our love for Him.

We want to spend time with people we love. We remember them and do thoughtful things. We think and speak fondly of them and feel happy and fortunate to have such treasured relationships. God loves us and desires, more than anything, to spend time with us. When we begin to love God in our current situation, He is able to navigate us through anything in ways we cannot on our own. In the presence of God, fear is moved and replaced with joy and peace. These are two of the many benefits of spending time with God.

Jesus coaches us to love God. Jesus brings us to the realization that we need God. **To be well, embracing God's way is essential.**

"Those who think they can do it on their own end up obsessed with measuring their own moral muscle but never get around to exercising it in real life. Those who trust God's action in them find that God's Spirit is in them—living and breathing God! Obsession with self in these matters is a dead end; attention to God leads us out into the open, into a spacious, free life. Focusing on the self is the opposite of focusing on God. Anyone completely absorbed in self ignores God, ends up thinking more about self than God. That person ignores who God is and what he is doing. And God isn't pleased at being ignored" (Romans 8:5-8).

Caring for Self

> Loving me points me to the God, Love, and Truth in me. —S.A.J.

In that love for God, we can embrace the second commandment and appreciate our self. God has commanded us to love ourselves. In Matthew 22:39, we see that caring for ourselves is necessary before we can authentically love others. Loving yourself is an extension of loving God. God made you for Himself. He values you highly! You are a custom-made, one-of-a-kind designer original. "He brought us to life using the true Word, showing us off as the crown of all His creatures" (James 1:18). **God's command: love what I gave you!**

God's love for us is without question. The Creator wants to love us, so open your heart and let His love flow in. As the love flows in, release the need to carry pain. Release the shame. Swing open the unforgivingness chamber within your heart and invite love in. Allow love to redress all wounds from the past. Now let that love flow into your mind. Be renewed fully through the energy of Jesus. Unhook all of your past and allow Him to re-hang it behind the protected helmet of salvation. Yield your imagination to Him to purge all of the negative scripts that continuously play. Let Him insert the truth of who you are. Allow His love to show you how valuable you are to Him. Now, honor that relationship by caring for yourself. Yield your future by allowing hope in your Primary Care giver to make you feel confident that He is with you no matter what. As you do this, you will begin to feel better. It will set the standard of care for how others are to care for you.

Do you remember the first time you held a newborn baby? Do you remember what a special moment that was? It was amazing how little and fragile the baby seemed. We realized this baby needed us and there was nothing we wouldn't do for this precious child. We needed to have the purest of everything. The baby needed pure air and chemical-free food, clothing, and ointments. This newborn child also needed a quiet, safe, and loving environment in which to grow. Think about it: once upon a time that baby was you! Just as special with the same needs and care. Many of us have lost sight of the fact that we are still the "baby." As adults, we need the purest of everything as well. We still need pure air, food, clothing, and ointments. A quiet, safe, and loving environment is needed for our healing, growth, and well-being. As adults, the caregiver role has shifted to us rather than remaining with our parents.

So it is the will of God for us to love and take care of ourselves. Our bodies house His Spirit and therefore, we must honor the presence of God within us. **This is the motivating factor for caring for ourselves: to honor God for the value He has placed on us and for being present within us.**

I am grateful to God for allowing me to be who I am. This gratitude lets me build a relationship based on mutual admiration and love that surpasses human comprehension. I did not always have this feeling. But now I see that how I love, care for, and treat myself and how I allow others to treat me is an act of worship. It is a 24-hour, seven-day-a-week process that ensures a peaceful, holistic existence. My way of living is governed by the demonstration and respect for this wonderfully predestined being, who is fully empowered to worship, praise, and make God proud. It feels so right.

> **A cheerful disposition is good for your health. —Proverbs 17:22**

Many of us go through life with the expectation that someone will come along and love us the way we want to be loved. We get disappointed as each person falls short of this unrealistic task. We attempt to treat others the way we want to be treated. Others can come close, but there is a place within us that only we can fill for ourselves. We must be an example, reflecting God's love by loving ourselves. How we respect, protect, nourish, and rest ourselves demonstrates our love and our value. Notice that caring for yourself does not mean having the largest, most extravagantly decorated home, the closet with the latest fashions, or the fine, expensive car. Oftentimes, these things disrupt our peace, produce shallow relationships, and place us in circles where we are not comfortable. Having possessions is not bad if we receive them on the path of obedience that God has designed for us. However, "things" do not symbolize loving ourselves as Christ commands.

I am convinced that loving myself is not easy. I am up close and personal with all my warts and past mistakes. I know where all my skeletons are buried. All my imperfections and shortcomings are labeled in flashing neon lights across my mind. When I do reluctantly forgive myself, I will never forget what I forgave myself for. With the enemy's help, I can relive it within seconds. Loving myself is so difficult that I would rather leave it to someone else. When I compare myself to others, I see even more of my imperfections.

We must remember that the most perfect person is perfectly imperfect! What perfects us is our wiring to God through Jesus Christ. We will never know perfection without primary care of God our Father. So it is sickening to attempt such a fate. I am lovable just as I am. Jesus proves that to me over and over again. My self-worth has little to do with me, and everything to do with Him who made me and decided who I should be. Loving my imperfect self is what allows me to be less critical, more accepting, and more loving of others. Love is fruitful. Love is planted within me and then gets pollinated from me into the life of others. Authentic love is sourced from God.

Caring for Others

Loving others is also a command from God according to Matthew 22:39. When we embrace God's love for ourselves, we are then to reflect His love to others. It is almost impossible to love others on a consistent basis without an understanding of our relationship to God.

> We must seek the Lord for love in each relationship, according to I Corinthians 13:1-8,13.

As we accept our relationship with God, we become the church, which is known as the Body of Christ. It is also referred to as the Kingdom of God. The church is not the brick and mortar that we see. The church is the collective group of people who have accepted Christ. They are pursuing wellness through the primary care of God and transitioning from their old lifestyle into a new one. The church often appears dysfunctional because there are millions of individuals, all flowing in love and moving toward wellness and the unique work that they were created to do. The path of wellness for each individual is different. Becoming well may be a mind, body, or spirit issue for each person. The brick-and-mortar church is the place where we go to honor God collectively. Our personalized work is what God would like us to do for the greater good of everyone. The relationship we now have with God is the love we reflect to others. Walking in love is the key to being well.

These interdependencies help make us complete. The family, the core structure established by God to sustain our earthly existence, is essential. The brokenness of the family unit is a major contributor to the dysfunction within our diseased culture. However, love is a commandment. We are instructed in Scripture to love one another the way Christ loves us. "This is how everyone will recognize that you are my disciples—when they see the love [and care] you have for each other" (John 13:34-35). As our relationship with God grows, we will learn that loving others is not a cookie-cutter process. Each of us has our own way of loving others. Our love is often directed in certain ways and may be closely tied to our purpose in life. An awareness and concern about things, such as the environment, our neighbors, our schools, food supply, and the world, all remind us that life is bigger than us as individuals. As we pray, we must consider the welfare of others, especially those who do not know Jesus, his healing, restorative power, and the freedom that makes us well. As we move toward developing the discipline of love for others, we will soon see how overwhelming it is if not for the help of God. We will never get it totally right, but we must move toward the goal and see each day as an opportunity to reflect God's love within the Kingdom and on the battlefield.

> And this I pray, that your love may abound yet more and more in knowledge and in all judgment; that ye may approve things that are excellent; that ye may be sincere and without offence till the day of Christ. Being filled with the fruits of righteousness, which are by Jesus Christ, unto the glory and praise of God. —Philippians 1:9-11 (KJV)

How Do We Love?

When we let Jesus into our hearts and believed in Him as our Lord and Savior, love was made perfect in us. We no longer have to look for it. We don't "go to" God because He is already with us and within us.

Loving family, friends, associates, strangers, and enemies—we are capable of loving all of them with God's help. It is easy to love the lovable. God helps us love the not so lovable. Scripture teaches us that love is foundational for all that we do. We gain strength as we love. If we demonstrate love on our own strength, which many of us do, it can make us weak. This is the Apostle Paul's description of love in action as written in I Corinthians 13:

> "If I speak with human eloquence and angelic ecstasy but don't love, I'm nothing but the creaking of a rusty gate. If I speak God's Word with power, revealing all his mysteries and making everything plain as day, and if I have faith that says to a mountain, 'Jump,' and it jumps, but I don't love, I'm nothing. If I give everything I own to the poor and even go to the stake to be burned as a martyr, but I don't love, I've gotten nowhere. So, no matter what I say, what I believe, and what I do, I'm bankrupt without love. Love never gives up. Love cares more for others than for self. Love doesn't want what it doesn't have. Love doesn't strut, doesn't have a swelled head, doesn't force itself on others, isn't always 'me first,' doesn't fly off the handle, doesn't keep score of the sins of others, doesn't revel when others grovel, takes pleasure in the flowering of truth, puts up with anything, trusts God always, always looks for the best, never looks back, but keeps going to the end. Trust steadily in God, hope unswervingly, love extravagantly. And the best of the three is love."

> He who does not love has not become acquainted with God for God is love. —I John 4:8 (AMP)

So how do we think of love in the context of living all day every day? Remember that love never changes. Love is constant. We disconnect from love by our thoughts and actions. Love never disconnects from us. Love is unconditional. So wherever we are, whatever we are doing, as we stay in the moment, our meditation should be: "Lord, help me to know your perfection in this moment." So whether that moment finds you facing a difficult situation with your boss or an enemy, enjoying your grandbaby, taking an exam, at a job interview, or having a discussion with your medical doctor, we can stay in love and know peace in the moment. Let's discuss other areas that might challenge our new loving discipline.

Love in the Kitchen

Well people demonstrate a lot of love in the kitchen. I personally have never liked to cook. It is always a surprise when people hear me say this; after all, I do practice holistic nutrition and my meals are delicious. But what keeps me in the kitchen is this: food made with love is powerful. I am in love with my Owner, and as a result, I love me and am able to love the people He has entrusted me to love. I want to strengthen and encourage them all. **One of the most powerful positions in the home and within an organization is the individual responsible for feeding people.** This person is a healer or destroyer depending on the type of food they serve, and reinforces and encourages the well-being of those entrusted to him or her if they serve healthy food. The body reacts to the energy, or lack thereof, in food.

Meals that have been prepared with ingredients that are weeks or months away from a garden or farm will provide less energy than fresh foods that are within days from their harvest date. Meals prepared with foods that have been rehydrated and preserved in order to prevent perishing will also have less energy.

Food preparation is an act of love. Family meals should be a team effort. The entire household should be involved in some way with putting a loving meal together as often as possible. In my household over the years, we have managed to maintain at least one meal together each day. When that is not possible, we brown bag. Carrying food from home serves many purposes. Yes, it saves money, yet it also packs an emotional connection to the loving, peaceful place where we live.

Love at Work

One of the issues with work life is that many of us find ourselves doing jobs that do not give us the ability to grow or use all of our skills and expertise. Work environments don't always pay people to think. It is actually the opposite: we are paid to think little and do a lot. As a result, a good portion of a typical day is connected to work-related activities: preparing to go, actually going, doing the work, and then leaving. Leadership training is not always given to company leaders who are asked to meet demands beyond their control. People handle their frustration related to work differently and we can find ourselves in high-stress and sometimes emotionally toxic environments.

Love at work, in most cases, is not straightforward. We need to know God's Word and the leadership of the Holy Spirit to assist us with how to reflect His love in a work environment. He will help us put our jobs in perspective. Think of your job as being your current Kingdom assignment. You don't get up in the morning to go to work. You get up in the morning to live! Work is a part of your life. It is important to pursue fulfillment outside of work through family projects, volunteering, church groups, hobbies, and other activities.

Our love at work is demonstrated in how we handle our responsibility. Do we go the extra mile? We see love played out in how we handle difficulties and conflict. We love through our trustworthiness, dependability, calm and gentle spirit, and by offering words of encouragement to others. We do a lot of forgiving. We respect the rank of our employer even though the individual holding that office may not be lovable.

Love at Church

Perfect love casts out fear. —I John 4:18 (NKJV)

When I was a young adult, success was defined by the diseased culture. Because I was well trained in the political nature of organizations, it was a struggle for me to embrace church membership. As a child who was raised in church settings, I witnessed a lot of jockeying for position and power. I was afraid to get involved. At that point I had a heartfelt conversation with God. I asked Him if it would be possible for me to please Him without being a part of a church. I wanted a relationship with God, but I wanted to avoid the others that He had brought into the Kingdom. So the common sense questions came: What is the church? And does Scripture say that I must be a part of a church?

The church is God's reflection within each of us. We reflect His truth, which makes us one—one body, many members. "So we, being **many,** are one body in Christ, and every one **members** one of another" (Romans 12:5, KJV). Christ is the head of the body (Colossians 1:18). We gather to worship and remember Christ's sacrificial death through Holy Communion and how he stood in our place so we could reconnect with God. Therefore, "we fellowship one with another" (I John 1:7, KJV). Larry Lea in his book *Could You Not Tarry One Hour?* suggests an appropriate prayer: "Lord, plant me in my local church and allow me to be a contributing, functioning, healthy part of that body."

So I obeyed and became a part of a church. That one act of obedience despite my fears put me on a path of right relationship with God. I now am a part of a population that has a loving relationship with the Father. None are perfect, but all seek to know Him in His perfection and desire for us. We are imperfectly linked, yet made lovingly functional because of our bond to Christ.

Love with Family

Loving family can be difficult because there are so many members of the family who reflect each other's behaviors. This includes how they handle problems and stress, their lifestyles and attitudes. As a result, conflicts are often taken to higher degrees of intensity. In the absence of a mediator, relationships become estranged and ties are broken beyond repair. Families seem more vulnerable to the warfare for wellness. Family is the conduit for love. We have our guard down and have an expectation that our family will care, share, and be accepting of us in our triumphs and imperfections. These expectations—some realistic, some not so—are used by the enemy to break down families. P.M. Smith says, "The family is God's first unit of government." It was established in a theocratic environment and is sustainable. When we attempt to be family outside of the Kingdom of God, we are made vulnerable to poor communication, competition, jealousy, disrespect, unforgivingness, and other foolish behaviors.

When I was a child, my parents engaged the entire household in family prayer. Dad's motto: "The family that prays together stays together." This also reminds me of Christ's promise, "For where two or three are gathered together in my name, there am I in the midst of them" (Matthew 18:20, KJV). Praying daily on issues that arise is the answer to loving family.

If you are not in a Christ-like relationship with your family, you must take the high road. Your personal prayer life and knowledge of God's Word are key. You should be able to reflect the love of God and His demeanor in both good and bad times. Your day-to-day life will give God the opportunity to reach your family, not by force or condemnation, but through authentic love. You could be the instrument in God's hands.

Love with Enemies and the Difficult

It is impossible to love the unlovable without an intervention from God who desires to use us to show His love to them. We are ambassadors of His love. We do good things for our enemies because God does good things for them. He lets the sun shine on everyone. God has provided instructions and promises to us for relating to our enemies. For example, "So let's not allow ourselves to get fatigued doing good" (Galatians 6:9). He will make your enemies to be at peace with you (Proverbs 16:7) or He will prepare a table for you in the presence of your enemies (Psalm 23:5). We are not perfect and we will not be able to perfectly execute God's will in everything we do. Jesus covers our imperfection with his perfection, which makes our wellness possible.

The discipline of pursuing primary care is essential to wellness. We are lovers. Practice the art of avoiding hate, loving our Maker, loving what our Maker made, and loving who our Maker has made. See your reflection in others and, miraculously, love shows you what to do next. Know that acts of kindness and tough love for correction and safety are all a part of the discipline of pursuing primary care as seen in Scripture.

It is easy to love the lovable. God helps us love the not so lovable.
—S.A.J.

Checklist for Discipline One: Pursue Primary Care
According to Matthew 22:37–39

Primary Care	Phase I	Phase II	Results
Loving God	Make God a priority. Identify idols that replace God. Pray and read the Bible daily.	Schedule time with God in your daily routine. Ask God to help you love Him. Pray and obey.	Peace Elimination of chronic stress. Less drama, more benefits.
Loving Self	Thank God daily for creating you. Begin by listing gifts and talents God has given to you.	Realize that God has invested Himself in you. Ask God to help you see your value.	Less drama, a sense of well-being. Accepting yourself.
Loving Others	Pray for wisdom and understanding on how to love others.	Become less critical. See the good in people.	Serving as unto God.

 Because God cares for me and I care for Him, I can care for others and myself.

 Primary care is God's love moving in and through me as I pursue Him.

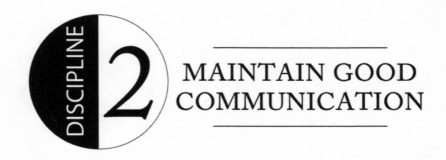

MAINTAIN GOOD COMMUNICATION

> Evening, and morning, and at noon, will I pray, and cry aloud: and he shall hear my voice. —Psalm 55:17 (KJV)

In order to know wellness as God intends, we must stay in communication with Him. This is called prayer. We are wired to pray. As a reflection of Himself, God made sure that our connection to Him would remain essential to our well-being. One of the many names of God is Jehovah, which means the "grace of God dwelling with His people." It is what makes our relationship with the all-powerful, all-knowing God up close and personal. Prayer is simply focusing the mind and opening up to a conversation with God. Prayer is effective when we believe that God exists and our relationship with Him is based on Jesus Christ. Prayer is a privilege of God's children to come to the one who was, is, and always will be our Primary Caregiver. The Father has an expectation that we will come to Him with everything! I am convinced that lack of prayer leads to many unnecessary issues. Prayer has been scientifically proven to impact our immune system in a positive way, according to Drs. Tolson and Koenig in *The Healing Power of Prayer*. Many Scriptures encourage us to pray at all times.

- ❖ Jesus told the disciples a story showing that it was necessary for them to pray consistently. (Luke 18:1)
- ❖ Evening, and morning, and at noon, will I pray, and cry aloud: and he shall hear my voice. (Psalm 55:17, KJV)
- ❖ He kneeled upon his knees three times a day, and prayed, and gave thanks before his God, as he did aforetime. (Daniel 6:10b, KJV)
- ❖ [Jesus] went up into a mountain apart to pray. (Matthew 14:23)

❖ Watch ye therefore, and pray always, that ye may be accounted worthy to escape all these things that shall come to pass, and to stand before the Son of man. (Luke 21:36, KJV)

❖ Pray without ceasing; in spirit and in truth. (I Thessalonians 5:17; John 4:23-24, KJV)

In other words, we are told to have a **life of prayer**. We are instructed to pray three times each day. What about praying nonstop? You may think: how can it be possible to pray at all times and ever get anything accomplished? Praying constantly does not mean head bowed down, hands together, and eyes closed. It does mean that we live life consciously in the presence of God and are open to His will for us. This keeps us strong, connected, in love, at peace, and able to live well and productively.

A prayer life is one that grows and matures over time as we develop the discipline of prayer. Getting started is difficult for some people. Many do not know what to pray. Hearing the eloquent prayers of others can be intimidating. It seems as if some people have become experts in prayer formulas, techniques, or programs. According to Matthew 6:5-13 (MSG, KJV), Jesus taught his disciples to pray with simplicity and discretion:

"And when you come before God, don't turn that into a theatrical production either. All these people making a regular show out of their prayers, hoping for stardom! Do you think God sits in a box seat? Here's what I want you to do: Find a quiet, secluded place so you won't be tempted to role-play before God. Just be there as simply and honestly as you can manage. The focus will shift from you to God, and you will begin to sense His grace. The world is full of so-called prayer warriors who are prayer-ignorant. They're full of formulas and programs and advice, peddling techniques for getting what you want from God. Don't fall for that nonsense. This is your Father you are dealing with, and He knows better than you what you need. With a God like this loving you, you can pray very simply. Like this: *Our Father who art in heaven, hallowed be thy name. Thy kingdom come, thy will be done in earth, as it is in heaven. Give us this day our daily bread. And forgive us our debts, as we forgive our debtors. And lead us not into temptation, but deliver us from evil. For thine is the kingdom, and the power, and the glory forever. Amen."*

Many of us know this prayer but have never stopped to consider this prayer as it was intended. Jesus provided a prayer outline for us to follow. Each phrase provides a powerful dialogue for us to pray to the Father now that we are in Christ.

Prayer	Meaning
Our Father who art in heaven, hallowed be thy name.	Praise and worship. Come into His courts with thanksgiving and praise, remembering the powerful names of God—God Almighty, Jehovah, Father, etc.—which are the foundations of our faith. Acknowledge our access to Him through the pure blood and sacrifice of Jesus the Christ.
Thy kingdom come, thy will be done in earth as it is in heaven.	Embrace the will of the Father in the world and in my life. I yield my desire because I trust Him and believe He knows best. I dwell in His Kingdom.
Give us this day our daily bread.	Petition for provision. Each day we believe that He will supply exactly what is needed, including knowledge and understanding as well as physical provisions, resources, and well-being.
And forgive us our debts, as we forgive our debtors.	Help us forgive all who have sinned against us. Petition for forgiveness of our sins as we turn in obedience to God's way.
And lead us not into temptation, but deliver us from evil.	Declare God's power and protection against Satan and his weapon—the diseased culture—for we have the full Armor of God (Ephesians 6:11).
For thine is the kingdom, and the power, and the glory forever. Amen.	Declare that God's Kingdom is where we live. He empowers us to live well. His love is our source of wellness always and forever.

As we mature in our prayer life, we can expand it to include other Scriptures to help us in our battle for wellness. A helpful tool in developing your prayer life is what I call a prayer framework, which contains activities of prayer that allow us to maintain good communication with God. These activities provide situational and practical ways to maintain our day-to-day relationship with the Father. This framework will help us live the instructions given by the Apostle Paul that tell us to "pray without stopping."

> Prayer is a privilege—not a burden. —D. James Kennedy

Common sense tells us that a prayer framework is not a very practical endeavor if it holds true to our traditional acts of prayer within the diseased culture. These traditional acts of prayer include short one-way conversations at morning and bedtime, grace at mealtimes, and prayer in times of trouble. We must see prayer as a 24/7 connection to God. It is life within the Kingdom. The atmosphere within the Kingdom is love, illuminated by the power of God. Our prayer keeps us plugged in, strengthened, and positioned in the presence of God. Life in the Kingdom is the realm in which "we live, and move, and have our being" (Acts 17:28, KJV). We need a prayer framework. Intelligent prayer is how we are spiritually nourished. In using this framework, our trinity must be involved. Scripture admonishes us to bless the Lord with our soul and all that is within. When we pray, our body, thoughts, imagination, subconscious, and emotions must be engaged.

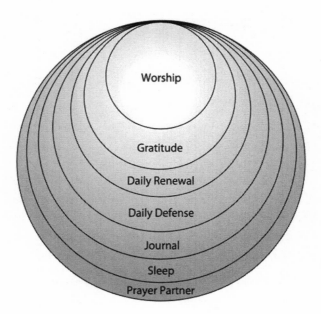

It is important that we connect to the God force in our lives several times a day. With this habit, our future has just been sealed for a path beyond what we can imagine. We do not have the capacity to see the total picture of our lives, but staying connected to God is essential. God can make the impossible possible.

> Prayer leaps over all barriers, stops at no distances and balks at no obstacles because it is in touch with the infinite resources of heaven.
> —Dr. M.R. DeHaan

Worship
Suggested Reading: Psalm 96-99, 104

Worshipping God is our best effort to hold Him in high regard. Above all others, we acknowledge His deity, greatness, power, and love in our lives. Worship is the connection we make through the Spirit and truth (John 4:24) to give glory to God our Father and the Lord Jesus Christ. In order to worship God, we must have chosen and received that new relationship with God through Jesus Christ. This relationship lets us have a renewed mind centered on God and a heart that has no unconfessed sin.

> Prayer helps us align our choices to what God wants.

Gratitude
A grateful heart fortifies our trinity. Thankfulness is the partner to worship. With gratitude we acknowledge what God has done, what He is doing, and what we know He will do based on His Word and all the promises He has made to His children. We are thankful for all His provisions and for the opportunity to acknowledge His goodness and mercy toward us. We are grateful that He is dependable, faithful, and committed to a relationship with us. Each of us can list those unique areas in our lives where God has blessed, protected, and helped us. We are full of so many answered prayers. We are reminded by Paul in his letter to the Philippians, "Do not be anxious about anything, but in every situation, by prayer and petition, with **thanksgiving**, present your requests to God" (Philippians 4:6, NIV). We are grateful that God's love never, ever fails.

> Enter into his gates with thanksgiving, and into his courts with praise: be thankful unto him, and bless his name. —Psalm 100:4, KJV

Daily Renewal

Suggested Reading: Psalm 103

It is difficult to heal when we are busy. But God is willing and able. To be renewed and refreshed every day, spend 15-30 minutes for prayer, Scripture meditation, breathing, and stretching. Jesus said, "Are you tired? Worn out? Burned out on religion? Come to me. Get away with me and you'll recover your life. I'll show you how to take a real rest. Walk with me and work with me—watch how I do it. Learn the unforced rhythms of grace. I won't lay anything heavy or ill-fitting on you. Keep company with me and you'll learn to live freely and lightly." (Matthew 11:28-30). It will seem awkward when we first attempt this mini-retreat for renewal, however, the benefit will encourage us to keep going. For many of my clients, the best time for daily renewal is just after work but right before reconnecting with family.

As of this writing, my father is 92 years young. For many years, he maintained three jobs in order to provide for his family. I have seen him extremely exhausted, and through prayer I have watched his restoration. Dad anoints himself with oil and lays before the Lord daily. When sickness appeared in his body, he constantly used prayer and supplication before the Lord and his health was restored. And Dad doesn't get sick very easily. There are few times when I have seen him sick—including a common cold.

For those who are in the Kingdom of God, we bear all the rights and privileges of being called His children and being able to call Him Father, our only Healer. We can go to Him, and He will give us His full attention!

> He heals all your diseases. —Psalm 103:3

Just for a few moments each day in prayer, use your imagination (putting it under the authority of the Holy Spirit) to lay your body before God and ask Him to reset it. Speak to every cell in your body, every organ, every thought, instructing them to yield to the Father. Then ask the Father to cleanse each of them, sweeping away the waste wherever it may be and allowing it to exit your body appropriately and in order. Release anger, stress, fear, and unforgivingness that may be inside you. Allow God to do a sweep of your emotions, thoughts, and imagination. Remember the work and the investment God has made in you and assure Him that you desire to complete your assignment. Receive complete wholeness delivered by the Christ. See in your mind the peace of God pouring into every cell, filling every organ, fully saturating your entire body like water into a sponge. And the peace of God, which surpasses every thought, will guard your hearts and your minds in Christ Jesus. Seal it with your faith and a grateful heart. Amen.

Daily renewal is a preventive strategy of the child of God in order to survive the warfare that is out to destroy us. This prayer prevents a build up of issues within our trinity that over time can surface as an ailment or disease. This practice is effective when used with the other disciplines. As we mature in this habit and our faith grows through our understanding of our provisions through Christ, we can work through chronic conditions and various illnesses.

> Heal me, O LORD, and I will be healed; save me, and I will be saved, for you are the one I praise. —Jeremiah 17:14 (NIV)

We must pray for healing and restoration, but God heals in the way He determines is best for us. It may not be an immediate healing. It could be healing through a medical procedure or through a behavioral change that He empowers us to make. We pray for guidance and flow with the healing process. Drs. Tolson and Koenig tell us, "You lock into the [healing] power [of God] through prayer. By praying to God and surrendering to Him, you allow God to activate the spiritual and physiological mechanisms that lead to wholeness and restoration."

> Prayer is helplessness casting itself on power.
> —Warren Wiersby

Daily Defense

Suggested Reading: Ephesians 6:10; I Peter 5:8-10

We discussed the importance of knowing your strengths and your weapons as a child and soldier of God. Scripture in Ephesians 6:10-11 encourages us: "God is strong, and he wants you strong. So take everything the Master has set out for you, well-made weapons of the best materials. And put them to use so you will be able to stand up to everything the Devil throws your way." As we go to God in prayer, we acknowledge the provisions He has made for us to be conquerors over the work of the enemy that is meant to discourage, deflect, and ultimately prevent us from completing our life's purpose. Just as we dress our physical bodies every day, we must also dress spiritually and mentally using the protective awareness as discussed in Scripture. For it is written, there is a natural [physical] body and a spiritual body (I Corinthians 15:44). As we pray and recite the many promises of God for protection, healing, and peace, we can be refreshed and feel safe and secure.

> The one concern of the Devil is to keep Christians from praying. He fears nothing from prayerless studies, prayerless work, prayerless religion. He laughs at our toil, mocks at our wisdom, but trembles when we pray.
> —Samuel Chadwick

Prayer has been scientifically proven to affect the immune system in a positive way. "But his delight is in the law of the LORD; and in His law doth he meditate day and night" (Psalm 1:2, KJV).

- ❖ Retreat every day for 15-30 minutes to perform prayer, meditation, breathing, and stretching.
- ❖ Offer up petitions and supplications for issues and concerns.
- ❖ Enjoy stress management through prayer.

> [Jesus said] This is what I want you to do: Ask the Father for whatever is in keeping with the things I've revealed to you. Ask in my name, according to my will, and He'll most certainly give it to you. Your joy will be a river overflowing its banks! —John 16:23-24

Journal

Having a journal as a part of our prayer framework can be a very valuable tool. A journal is a book, normally bound and blank, used exclusively for your time and study with the Father. Like prayer, journaling helps free the mind, giving you more capacity to handle other things. We journal to keep our prayer life organized and effective, as instructed in I Timothy 2. We are told to make our **requests** known, **pray for others**, and offer up **prayers of thanksgiving**. In our journal, we should designate a section for each of these categories according to I Timothy 2:1-4:

❖ **Prayer requests:** Make a list every day. Some will be repeated, and new requests will be noted. Include needs, problems, fears, worries, and stressors. Ask for guidance and peace with faith for the answer.

❖ **Prayers for others:** Also called intercessory prayers. List concerns and needs of people you know personally and those you do not. Include prayers for those lost without Christ, our nation, the sick, the widow or widower, etc.

Below is a list of examples of prayers for others:

- o Inconsiderate neighbor
- o Pastor and family and church leadership
- o Safety and favor for Dad at the nursing home
- o Tomorrow night's dinner guests
- o Traveling mercies for Patricia
- o The peace of Israel
- o The homeless and hungry children
- o Those living without Christ

❖ **Prayers of thanksgiving:** With a grateful heart, list those things you are thankful for. Include answered prayers and the smallest to the largest blessing of the day. (Philippians 4:8)

At the end of your journaling session, in prayer pass this list to the Father for His will to be done and believe that each item will have His personal attention. If you make these lists in the morning, it may be helpful to update those requests before bed. Again, this will free your mind and prevent restless sleep.

Sleep

Why is sleep a part of the prayer framework? Sleep is a prayer posture. It is a sacred time of fellowship and restoration with God the Father. It is the time when we yield our conscious selves with a grateful heart to Him for safekeeping and the subconscious is still. During sleep, God engages the human trinity to heal, reconcile, and restore, and the past, present, and future have no boundaries. Images of events, issues, fears, and people can converge into the same experience. In dreams, our realities and imaginations come together to bring about outcomes that would not have been possible if we were conscious. During sleep, the body repairs cells, burns fat, regulates hormones, and reduces inflammation.

> Don't you know he enjoys giving rest to those he loves?
> —Psalm 127:2

Sleep hygiene, or the promotion of good sleep habits, is good stewardship. Never watch television, have phone conversations, or use electronics in bed. This practice stimulates the brain and body. It sends a mixed message because the body is attempting to shut down, but the use of electronics does just the opposite. Many of us think that watching television in bed awake or leaving it on while asleep is harmless. But it is very dangerous for a child of God who wants to be well. When we are asleep, we have no filters and our subconscious is available to receive whatever it is exposed to. Some of my clients actually admit that their dreams include whatever is on television. The best way to rest the conscious and subconscious is to experience restful sleep in silence and darkness, which eliminates all opportunities for the subconscious to be engaged. Insomnia would be cured for many of us if we changed this one behavior.

Here are some other sleep hygiene tips that I have found to be helpful to my clients over the years, many of which are also recommended by the National Sleep Foundation:

- ❖ Go to bed and wake up on a regular schedule.
- ❖ Prepare your bedroom for sleep: darken the room, place a flashlight on your nightstand, make sure that your walking path to the bathroom is clear.
- ❖ Do not sleep with an electric blanket or electronics near your bed.
- ❖ Eat your last meal three hours before bedtime.
- ❖ Reduce disturbing noises with a fan or white noise machine.
- ❖ Reduce or eliminate caffeine and sugar consumption.
- ❖ Keep clutter off the bed.
- ❖ Do not eat or drink in bed.
- ❖ Introduce wind-down times for each person in your family to get quiet; dim the lights and turn off electronics, including cell phones.
- ❖ In your journal, make a list of everything on your mind that may cause restlessness: things to do, things to remember, concerns, and fears. Then pray.
- ❖ Have your evening prayers and place your consciousness in the presence of the Lord with a grateful heart.

Many of us are not aware of how abusive sleep deprivation is to the body. It affects the immune system and our ability to fight off viruses and other ailments. "If your whole family is short on sleep and one of you has a cold, you're more likely to pass the virus around," says Dr. Helene A. Emsellem, author of *Snooze . . . or Lose!* Not only that but your family's risk of type 2 diabetes increases with sleep deprivation, according to the Sleep and Circadian Research Group at Woolcock Institute of Medical Research in Sydney, Australia. The research group also found that sleep positively affects your body's ability to process sugar. According to a 15-year study published in 2007 at Stanford University, lack of sleep can also lead to obesity by changing the levels of the sleep hormones that regulate your blood sugar. Emsellem adds, "If you already have diabetes, not sleeping can make it difficult to control your weight, which will make your diabetes worse."

Staying up late and eating after 7:00 p.m. can also cause weight gain. A study from Northwestern Medicine discovered that late sleepers ingested 248 more calories daily, mostly at dinner and later in the evening. They consumed half as many fruits and vegetables, twice the fast food, and drank more full-calorie carbonated drinks than those who went to bed earlier.

For children of God, sleep is a time to yield and be still. We can then be draped totally with God's love. The subconscious is the seat of the Holy Spirit. Sleep is the opportunity to rest wholly before God. God promised His children sweet, peaceful, and safe sleep (Proverbs 3:24; Psalm 4:8).

Sample morning prayers

Good morning, Father. Good morning, Jesus. Good morning, Holy Spirit. I worship you today. I put you in your rightful place, below no other, for you and you alone are worthy. Forgive me for my sins. Thank you for all good and perfect gifts. Thank you for so many answered prayers. Thank you for the gift of this day, a day that I will never see again. Please guide me, lead me, and teach me in the path of righteousness according to your will that I might glorify the Father and make Him proud. We pray for our pastor and leaders that they might lead well. Thy kingdom come, Thy will be done on earth as it is in heaven. In Jesus' name. Amen.

Dear Father, I thank you for this day. I am your child, I am your property, and I am your tool. Because of you, I live, move, and have my being. Use me today to your satisfaction. Not my will, but your will, be done in Jesus' name. Amen.

This is the day that the Lord has made. Let us rejoice and be glad in it. Let us rejoice and be at peace in it. Let us rejoice and see God in it. Let us rejoice and think, move, eat, and rest in it. This is the day; this is the day that the Lord has made! Amen and amen!

Prayer Partner

A wise follower of Christ once shared that having a prayer partner was an extension of the fellowship of believers that is mentioned in Scripture. Jesus makes a promise in Matthew 18:20, "When two of you get together on anything at all on earth and make a prayer of it, my Father in heaven goes into action. And when two or three of you are together because of me, you can be sure that I'll be there." When two people commit to agree in prayer, they are proclaiming their faith and trust in God, who keeps His promises. Having a prayer partner also helps us remain accountable. It provides a mirror for us to see ourselves. A prayer partner helps us to pray for the good of others. We can gain a more global perspective on the needs of others and the movement of God.

> Pray for your brothers and sisters. Keep your eyes open. Keep each other's spirits up so that no one falls behind or drops out.
> —Ephesians 6:18

Ask the Father for a prayer partner. You will need His assistance to make sure that you make the right selection. Your prayer partner should be of the same gender and have an upstanding reputation of Christ-like behavior. Prayer partners should meet for prayer at least once each week, however, circumstances from time to time may warrant more meetings. Because of technology, our prayer partner can be located almost anywhere. E-mail, phone, video conferencing, and text messages can be used in order to successfully maintain your bond. I recommend short prayer times which make it easier to fit this new commitment into your lifestyle. Share your needs and concerns, then pray, with each person taking a turn.

On the topic of stress management, Dr. James F. Balch and Mark Stengler in *Prescription for Natural Cures* state, "The most powerful mind-body relaxation technique, in our opinion, is prayer. It offers an opportunity to communicate with the Creator and cast your doubts and cares upon Him.

> True prayer is a way of life, not just a case of emergency. —Unknown

This is the time to 'be still' and hear from God. Make prayer a daily habit, and it will help you relax and achieve a more healthful life."

God never promised a smooth ride through life. In the midst of every joyful or sorrowful circumstance, however, you will find love. As you exercise this prayer framework, you will come to realize that your day is a well-orchestrated path uniquely prepared for you. For in Him we live, move, and have our being (Acts 17:28, KJV). God presents and allows every opportunity, circumstance, and encounter. Our spiritual health is nourished and restored within this process of prayer.

 A prayer life is essential to God's plan for wellness.

 The prayer framework can help me build a life of prayer.

DISCIPLINE 3

BE INTENTIONAL ABOUT LIFE

> And we know that all things work together for good to them that love God, to them who are the called according to His purpose.
> —Romans 8:28 (KJV)

W hen we consider the idea of being a VIP to God and loved beyond measure, it is a wonderful feeling. Scripture indicates that we were created in order to reflect God's love and honor Him through our living. We also learn that each of us has been given a specific purpose to collectively influence the good of all. We are uniquely wired by God to Himself for a specific purpose. My purpose is a complement, not a competitor, with your purpose, as we are tools used by the hand of God to His end.

One of the challenges with this exciting revelation is that many of us have negative thoughts, opinions, and conversations with ourselves. It is such a habit that we are not aware of it and more than likely are in denial of it. We have a low bar for who we are and what we will accomplish in life. It is the tool of the enemy to make sure this is solidified within you. But this kind of thinking is a lie! I cannot tell you all of the benefits of knowing Scripture and the comfort in knowing the promises that the Father has made to us. It includes hope, expectation, and encouragement that speak to the spirit of man. If for no other reason, allocating the time to spend in God's Word becomes the authentic foundation and security for knowing who you really are. It gets to the very fiber of your peace, your confidence, and your well-being. When you understand and embrace God's Word, you gain insight as to how He operates and thinks. This insight supports the things that God intends for us, the promises and empowerment that come out of His Word, how He sees us individually, and our significance within His Kingdom.

Realizing our unique purpose is said to be the beginning of a new life. It is that "Oh wow!" experience that connects the dots. Dr. Viktor Frankl, a psychiatrist who wrote *Man's Search for Meaning,* states that "Man's search for meaning is the primary motivation in life . . . This meaning is unique and specific in that it must and can be fulfilled by him alone." Unlike animals, human beings are free to decide and to achieve goals and purposes. The absence of meaningful goals and purpose creates a void that will give rise to aggression, addiction, depression, and other self-destructive behaviors. Each of us, therefore, has a unique purpose or meaning in life. Dr. Frankl continues, "Our purpose is the personal dedication to a cause greater than ourselves." In other words, our purpose benefits the greater good and demonstrates our love for others.

We know from Scripture that Christ became a human named Jesus. There was an assignment attached to his life, which was to rebuild our connection to God (John 1:4). Without this assignment, there would have been no reason for him to have a body. "We are permanent personalities dwelling in temporary bodies," explain Drs. Tolson and Koenig. Now that we know we reflect the nature of God, we too have an assignment attached to our lives—our purpose for being. We read in Psalm 139:16-18 that before we had lived one day, our entire life was planned. This point of intent and purpose for our lives is laced throughout Scripture (Ephesians 2:8-10; Jeremiah 29:11).

Living on purpose is what we do and how we flow with the divine hand of God and His purpose for our lives. It is the point when we put our intelligence back in God's hands to bring forth the plan for restoring our health, making it a plan that is doable and personalized for each of us. It may or may not be totally conscious at this time. Know that the life you are living and the path you are on are layers of preparation for the fulfillment of your purpose. For example, parenting and other family experiences provide many opportunities for the Lord to expose and fine-tune some of the essentials for your work. Your marriage and your children are good and perfect gifts from the Lord (James 1:17, NIV). These gifts and your

83

stewardship toward them will not conflict with your purpose. Or you may have a job that you absolutely hate. Believe me when I say that this job is a necessary pit stop on the path to your purpose. As a result, you may realize your purpose but will not mature in it for several years. Take heart, it will all come together for the greater good of mankind and bring glory to God.

> Life's most urgent question is: 'What are you doing for others?'
> —Martin Luther King, Jr.

Patience, faith, and excitement are key attributes of people who are waiting to do more of their special work. In the fullness of time, your path will become clear. The fragments of all you have been exposed to and all that makes you *you* will come together.

Every Christian has the same identity. We are children of God, and there is a lifestyle associated with this. We have the same commission, or charge, that is laid out in Matthew 28:19-20, which reads:

> Go ye therefore, and teach all nations, baptizing them in the name of the Father, and of the Son, and of the Holy Ghost: Teaching them to observe all things whatsoever I have commanded you: and, lo, I am with you alway, even unto the end of the world. Amen. (KJV)

As we walk in obedience to this commission and to the great commandment—love God, ourselves, and others—that love permeates all we do. Our purpose, however, is a unique talent, gift, or assignment that each of has attached to our life in Christ.

> With your very own hands you formed me; now breathe your wisdom over me so I can understand you. —Psalm 119:73

Determining Your Purpose (Life's Meaning)

First, we must believe that there is a larger meaning for our lives. It is important that I make a distinction about purposeful living. All children of God have a common goal: obedience to God. That is the baseline for all of us who love Him. Each of us has been given a special assignment. Scripture explains that there is a map for your life. Before I had even lived one day on Earth, my life was laid out (Psalm 139:16).

Second, we must release ourselves from the influence of the diseased culture, which can make us want to be popular, rich, and famous apart from God's glory.

Finally, take some time and consider the following questions. Your answers can be very helpful toward the discovery of your purpose.

1. What are the things I do to help people that make them appreciative and thankful for my help? Do I feel fulfilled?

2. What helpful talents or gifts come naturally to me?

3. What task brings so much enjoyment that I lose track of time?

4. What subjects do I find interesting and exciting?

5. What are the ills of the world that make me angry that I want to help fix?

6. What training or education have I really enjoyed?

7. Which tasks or activities do I love to do?

8. What would I do if I knew I couldn't fail?

9. What service can I render in which payment is not a priority?

10. What experience in life (good or bad) has challenged me and allowed me to learn some things that have had a lasting, positive impact?

If you are like many of us, you may answer these questions knowing that you are in a job or on a career path that is not fulfilling. It may not fire your rockets, but it pays the bills and allows you to afford the creature comforts in life.

> A man's gift maketh room for him, and bringeth him before great men.
> —Proverbs 18:16 (KJV)

Many of us are afraid to admit that this situation exists in our lives. But the truth will set you free! And denial could be killing you. Knowing this does not mean you should turn in your resignation first thing in the morning. Your occupation may not be your life's purpose, but you can answer your calling through volunteer work or part-time ministry. For example, Jesus was a carpenter (Mark 6:3) but becoming our Savior was his purpose. The Apostle Paul was a tentmaker by trade (Acts 18:3) but being a pastor and leader was his purpose. You cannot accomplish your purpose on your own. There are some questions you can begin asking God, letting Him know you're seeking knowledge and an understanding of your divine purpose. Once this is done, all of the answers to the above questions will begin to reveal a pattern that is distinctive to you. Some of them are stepping stones, and some are detours that might have taken you off track for a while.

As our purpose becomes clearer, the enemy of God will not make it easy for you to be successful with your work. Discouragement and opposition may come from some very unexpected places. However, we must hold on to the Word of God and obey His commands that we know to be true. The Apostle Paul says, "We pray that you'll live well for the Master, making him proud of you as you work hard in His orchard. As you learn more and more how God works, you will learn how to do your work. We pray that you'll have the strength to stick it out over the long haul—not the grim strength of gritting your teeth but the glory-strength God gives" (Colossians 1:10-11).

The Seven Disciplines will help us remain well and available to flow with the Father as He leads. The stages of our unique path will illuminate your purpose in the fullness of time.

Work-life balance

We discussed walking in love at work and how the leadership of the Holy Spirit will help us put our work in perspective. While important, employment represents a small portion of life overall, yet it seems to overshadow and impact everything we do or don't do. There is a saying: "We work to live. We shouldn't live to work." And yet within the diseased culture, life seems to revolve around work. As a result, this culture can bleed heavily into our lifestyles.

According to Center for Economic and Policy Research reports, United States employers are not required to provide paid vacation time or paid holidays. We also trail far behind many other countries in our maternity leave policies. Yet despite our work ethic, we are no less susceptible to economic collapse and recession, and it ends up costing us our health and well-being.

We can pray to God to help us improve our individual work-life balance situations. As we seek our individual intended purposes, we must establish boundaries to keep ourselves balanced and well. Here are some limitations you can set for yourself to give you greater work-life balance:

- ❖ Everyday I rise to live, not to go to work. My Kingdom life includes work. Work is one item on the list of things to do in the day.
- ❖ Before and after work, I manage my time to make sure that I do not overextend myself.
- ❖ I will not sacrifice health or family due to pressure and stress associated with work.
- ❖ I don't have to have all the answers at work. I will seek help from the Father for guidance and peace.
- ❖ My place of work is my assigned vineyard. I am a good steward. I pray for my employer, coworkers and our relationships.
- ❖ My attitude should reflect that of a diligent worker.
- ❖ I do not have to live in fear about my job. No change can happen unless my Father permits it. God is my source.

A Helpful Prayer

Father, you are holy and intentional about everything, including me. Thank you. Psalm 139 assures me that I have a purpose for living. I want to clearly become aware of my purpose. There is no other reason for me to live! At this point in my life, your will is my will. I am yielded and still. Help me to see the dots connect as my life's assignment becomes clearer. Thank you for making me whole and preparing me for this work. Help me to appreciate each day you give, the path you have set before me, the relationships, responsibility, provisions, and territory. Thank you for wellness in the Kingdom, for your glory in Jesus' name. Amen.

And we know that all things work together for good to them that love God, to them who are the called according to His purpose.
—Romans 8:28 (KJV)

 God has a special assignment for me for the greater good.

 Being well makes me available to complete that assignment.

USE COMMON SENSE

> I've written to warn you about those who are trying to deceive you. But they're no match for what is embedded deeply within you—Christ's anointing, no less! You don't need any of their so-called teaching. **Christ's anointing teaches you the truth** on everything you need to know about yourself and him, uncontaminated by a single lie. Live deeply in what you were taught. —I John 2:26-27

Based on common sense, we know that we need a relationship with God. We need to think and make good decisions. Early on in this book, we discussed common sense and what it means to have it. We defined common sense as making rational decisions based on what we know to be true. Common sense is a mental ability provided by God to each of us so we can think and exercise the gift of choice. We also discussed that in order to use common sense, we have to know the truth, which is God. Jesus said, "I am the way, the **truth**, and the life" (John 14:6). The Holy Spirit is referred to as the "Spirit of **Truth**." We know that our body is the temple of the Holy Spirit, meaning the Spirit lives within us and reflects the truth of God. In the Kingdom, the Spirit of Truth is with us forever according to John 14:16-17. That truth is always available to provide what we need to know in order to use common sense.

Another dimension to using common sense is presented by Dr. Elson Haas in his book *Staying Healthy with the Seasons*. Dr. Haas suggests that common sense is prevention at two levels. The first is called "avoidance" of what we know to cause harm, like alcohol, drugs, and smoking. The second level of prevention is the use of "positive action" which means having good behaviors on a regular basis that keep us healthy and prevent chronic disease.

These behaviors include physical exertion, healthy eating, healthy thoughts, self-education, and awareness.

In order to use common sense, we must get to know God through His map for our lives—His Word. Three steps make it possible:

1. We must study God's Word so that we will know the truth. Knowledge of His Word also allows us to pray intelligent prayers that complement His will for us. (II Timothy 2:15, Luke 11:1)

2. We must think about the truth and use it to measure all circumstances in life. (Psalm 33:4)

3. Based on what we know to be true and how a situation stacks up against the truth, we make the right decision. (Psalm 43:3)

The enemy's strategy is to make us too busy to think.

Only mature and well-exercised intelligence can save you from falling into gullibility (I Corinthians 14:20-25). When we were living outside the Kingdom of God, we had become a people who stopped thinking. We went along for the ride as opposed to being actively engaged in the process of living well. We gave the job of thinking over to someone else. The herd mentality—whatever the majority does—is what we do. There is little time to search for the truth, for thinking and making decisions. The enemy's strategy is to make us too busy. It is critical to his plan that we run out of time every day and never seem to get enough done. As a result, we feel unproductive and become more unorganized, feeling unworthy, and we are forced to go with the flow and with what seems right. We can also become disruptive within the ranks of the Kingdom when we begin to live out what we think instead of living life on God's terms, which keeps us fully engaged in battle. The Book of Wisdom warns us of going with the way that seems right, but the end is destruction (Proverbs 14:12). As a result, many relationships, organizations, churches, and governments suffer. I agree with Paul writing to the Christians in Corinth about Christ, "Ignorance of God is a luxury you can't afford in times like these" (I Corinthians 15:34).

Now that we are on a wellness path, we want to know the truth. We seek the truth. As soldiers in Christ's army, we must learn to manage all the resources that God has assigned to us. This includes time and life, health and strength, time and money, family and friends, and natural resources. We manage our resources based on what is important to us.

Time is a priceless resource that often gets misused or stolen. It is listed twice because it is an overarching resource in life and is an indicator of how we use money. Managing time is critical. Regaining control of our time starts with understanding that time is a gift and must be allocated properly. We all have been granted 24 hours each day. Yet some of us seem to get more out of our time than others. How we allocate each hour determines how well we will become. Go to Appendix B in the back of this book and complete the time log for a typical weekday and a weekend day. After you have completed the time log, what truths have you discovered about the use of your time? How much time is allocated to relaxing with the television or surfing the Web? Know that church service and doing good are not replacements for prayer and study time with the Lord. God is the power behind your church service and acts of kindness. We recharge through prayer and reading His Word to gain the strength to serve and know the truth.

Jesus had a very demanding ministry and twelve very needy students. In the midst of that, he set an example by praying early in the morning to the Father who set His day on course. As a result, his days were amazingly productive. Wanting to know how to do that, his students asked him to teach them how to pray. He taught them to pray "Thy kingdom come, thy will be done on earth as it is in heaven" (Matthew 6:10). In other words, "Let your spirit come to earth and dwell within me as it does in heaven." **Spending time with God every day allows His priorities to become our priorities.** Larry Lea wrote two effective prayers for time management on God's terms, "Lord, please fix my work habits. Help me to not be slothful or a workaholic, I need balance." The second is "Holy Spirit, help me to have a high quality, consistent, daily personal prayer life and time in the Word for fellowship daily with Jesus."

What is important to us is also important to the Father. Knowing the Father through His Word is the ammunition for soldiers to line up their behaviors and approach life within God's will. As a result, soldiers stay well. The Book of Wisdom also encourages us to "commit thy works unto the Lord, and thy thoughts shall be established" (Proverbs 16:3, KJV).

Common sense indicates that spending time every day in fellowship with Jesus is essential for fighting the wellness battle based on the truth.

Luke 15:11-23 tells us the story of a young son who lived with his father and brother. The family estate had great wealth. This young son informed his dad that he no longer wanted to live according to the way he had been raised or follow the path made for him to be well and great among the people. Leaving with his inheritance and freedom in hand, he enlisted in the popular culture to the fullest extent. Without the leadership and wisdom of his father, he fell into hard times and sunk very low into poverty of spirit, mind, and body. Finally finding himself starving, eating from an animal's bowl, he began to use common sense. He remembered the truth. He reflected on the goodness, provision, and real freedom that he had so taken for granted. He walked away from his hard life and returned humbly to his dad and asked for forgiveness. Then he was restored, which brought the father much joy.

Knowing the truth and going another way is rebellion against God our Father. It will not keep us well and can be very painful. Obedience to God and His way is common sense. Therefore, wellness is common sense, a gift God bestows upon His children.

Train me in good common sense; I'm thoroughly committed to living your way. Before I learned to answer you, I wandered all over the place, but now I'm in step with your Word. —Psalm 119:66-67

 Common sense is based on the truth, and God is truth.

 Wellness is common sense.

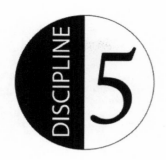

ESTABLISH A SACRED PLACE TO LIVE

A s soldiers in God's Kingdom, we must draw lines around our territory so we can restore our trinity daily. The place where we live physically is also Kingdom territory.

As you read this information about improving your living environment, please consider the changes to be made very carefully. Some of these changes must be implemented gradually. The fastest way to disrupt the peace you already enjoy is to go home and make a list full of proclamations without explanation or buy-in from key family members.

> In the Kingdom of God, love is the atmosphere in which we live.
> —S.A.J.

We can review many Scriptures that clearly demonstrate our Trinitarian nature and the impact that each attribute has on the whole person. Take a look at the following table of Scripture references. These Scriptures reinforce our need for a relationship with a God who understands our personal trinity and how to keep us well.

> Live well, live wisely, live humbly.
> —James 3:13

Spirit	Mind	Body
Love: Rom. 5:8; I John 4:16	**Love:** John 15:9-10; Rom. 12:9-13	**Love:** John 3:16; Romans 5:5
Faith: Rom. 12:3; Heb. 11:3	**Faith:** Eph. 3:12; Eph. 6:16; I Thess. 5:24	**Faith:** II Cor. 5:7; Eph. 6:16
Peace: I Tim. 6:6; Heb. 13:20-21	**Peace:** John 14:27	**Peace:** Prov. 16:7; James 3:18
Power: Eph. 1:17-19; I Tim. 2:7	**Well-being:** Rom. 8:39	**Rest, Comfort:** II Cor. 1:3-7
Purpose: Jer. 29:11; Eph. 2:22	**Purpose:** Ps. 139:16-17; I Thess. 4:11-12	**Purpose:** Ps. 139
Joy: Neh. 8:10; Ps. 16:11	**Emotions:** Rom. 5:1-2; Rom. 12:14-19	**Prayer:** Eph. 6:18
Values: Ps. 1:1; Ps. 26:3-12; John 15:5	**Character, Truth:** Eph. 4:22; Col. 3:9-10	**Head:** Eph. 6:17
Humility: Prov. 16:19	**Truth, Common Sense:** Prov. 13:15-16	**Hearing:** Prov. 15:31
Confidence: I John 5:14	**Attitude:** Prov. 17:22; Gal. 5:22-23	**Speech:** Prov. 10:20; Prov. 16:13,24; Eph. 4:29; II Tim. 2:16-17
Strength: Eph. 3:16	**Knowledge/Wisdom:** Prov. 16:20-21; Col. 2:3; Heb. 4:12	**Hands:** I Tim. 2:8
Goodness, Mercy: Ps. 23:6	**Self-control:** Prov. 15:28; Prov. 16:20; Eph. 4:26; James 1:19	**Eyes:** II Kings 6:17; Prov. 15:30
Patience: Ps. 37:7-9; Gal. 6:9	**Thoughts & Direction:** Prov. 15:22; Prov. 16:9; Col. 3:2	**Helper, Executor:** Eph. 1:13-14
Health: Ps. 42:11; Ps. 43:5	**Imagination:** II Cor. 10:4-6	**Protector:** Eph. 6:11; I Tim 6:12
Worship: Ps. 104	**Prayer:** Eph. 1:16; I Thess. 5:17	**Worship:** I Cor. 3:16; I Cor. 6:19-20; Eph. 3:14-15
	Hope: Col. 1:27	**Work:** I Thess. 3:10; James 1:27
	Gratitude: Ps. 100:4-5; Eph. 5:18-20	**Affliction:** Rom. 5:3
	Health: Eph. 4:23	**Fitness:** Acts 17:28; Rom. 12:1
		Death: II Cor. 5:8; Col. 3:3-4; I Thess. 4:14-16
		Walk: Eph. 5
		Health: James 5:16; III John 1:2

At a reception, I chatted with a nice gentleman who, after finding out the nature of my work, began to describe how he and his wife lived a very holistic life. He proceeded to use a mental checklist to describe his lifestyle. He mentioned their diet, his exercise regimen, sleep habits, and work philosophy. On his relationship with God through Jesus Christ, he stated, "My wife has that covered. She is extremely spiritual and starts every morning by going to church. It is not a formal service; she just likes to go there to pray." This man practiced wellness as defined by the diseased culture. He does not have his own relationship with Jesus Christ. He knows of Christ, but he does not know Christ. He had a portion of the disciplines but lacked the foundation on which to sustain a wellness lifestyle over time. On the other hand, I thought of his wife and how nice it would be if she found a place at home where she could have her morning prayers and get centered. She has an admirable custom, but a time may come when going out every day is not possible. This could be disruptive to her well-being if she feels that effective connection with God is not possible if she does not get out.

Home is our healing station. It is a **sacred place**, a reflection of all that we are and all that we think we can do and be in the world. It is a region in the Kingdom of God. A home does not have to be a mansion or have every toy and gadget known to man. It is not based on the market value or whether it has brick or aluminum siding. It can be a mobile home, an apartment, a dormitory room, a barracks, a homeless shelter, under an overpass, public housing, or a hotel room. You enter into a space with your peace. The question to ask yourself is "What is needed here in order for me to live in this space as God would have me live?" In this space, God's presence reigns, your peace is nourished, and your well-being is maintained.

Our sacred place is a cocoon for healing, growth, development, rest, relaxation, and renewal. It is a safe place, void of predators, toxins, and negative energies. Most of all, it is a controlled exposure to the diseased culture, including sensory overload from electronic devices. Jesus spent a lot of time in the homes of those who would follow him. Being in someone's home can reveal a lot about his or her values, character, and health. When we step out of our living space, we should be whole and prepared for each day. Once your sacred place is established, there will be some days when you will run off the battlefield of the world to the peace and healing that awaits you at home. So how do we configure a home environment that supports wellness as a lifestyle?

There are five things that build a special healing environment for each of us:
1. Good communication with all household members
   o Understanding of value system
   o Schedules and necessary routines
2. Clean air environment
3. Atmosphere
   o Colorful and peaceful

          o   Healing chambers

4. Organization

          o   Creating boundaries for each function

          o   Controlling clutter

5. Maintenance

Good Communication with All Household Members

First, develop a set of family values. These values can be written and discussed so all members of the household can fully embrace what they believe, how they operate, and how they choose to live. Values help us define who we are. Positive messages on plaques, on the refrigerator, or in artwork around the house provide reinforcement of our values. Here are some examples I have used:

Peace, this is what we choose every day.

The just shall live by faith. (Hebrews 10:38)

We walk by faith and not by sight. (II Corinthians 5:7)

Every word is a gift to the hearer. (Ephesians 4:29)

Friends are flowers in life's garden.

Happiness is being married to your best friend.

With God, all things are possible. (Matthew 19:26)

Never let the sun go down on your anger. (Ephesians 4:26)

Second, establish a way for the household to maintain effective communication. A household calendar is effective in planning and supporting one another. Create a family prayer life by setting aside a date and time for prayer and Bible reading. Establish a mealtime schedule and determine roles and responsibilities for the meal. From shopping to meal preparation to cleaning up, all of these tasks should be rotated. The benefit of rotating is that each person has an appreciation for the effort required to complete a task. Establish emergency procedures in case of fire or other calamity. For your children, build a community support system. Who are the trusted individuals in your circle who can stand in for you during a time of need?

Also establish standard family meetings where all family members can gather to discuss or resolve issues, such as family projects/vacation, spring cleaning, academic support, etc. One hour is the maximum time that should be allotted for this meeting. One hour is something everyone can plan around. An agenda with topics can be listed and given out prior to the meeting. This creates a structure so the meeting won't run overtime. Studies show that attendance, attentiveness, and cooperation are much better in meetings that are planned and start and end on time. Any family member can call a family meeting if circumstances warrant it. When my daughter was a little girl, she would occasionally call family meetings. Her issues (e.g., allowance, desire for a pet, sleepovers) were very important to her and thus important to us. When family members know there is a way to be heard and have their requests addressed, peace and calm can be maintained in the home.

Clean Air Environment

In the home, we must have a clean air environment. Although many of us have incorporated healthy eating and exercise into our lives, few of us have taken steps to reduce the number of pollutants, toxins, and other disruptors we are exposed to on a daily basis. It is impossible to fully control our environment, but we can become more aware of the toxins we can control and take action to consciously avoid them. Doing so is essential for maintaining a healthy immune system and quality living.

There is a branch of medicine called environmental medicine that seeks to increase scientific understanding of the health risks posed by contaminants at home, in the workplace, and in the ambient environment. It is not normal to have five or six colds a year, a runny nose in the winter, or recurring ear infections. The chemicals in our homes that compromise our immune systems may cause these illnesses.

Studies have revealed a stay-at-home parent has a near 50 percent higher chance of getting cancer than those who work outside the home. Many of our households have very high toxicity levels. Our carpeting, furniture, cleaning products, and insecticides are all sources of pollutants in our homes. The most toxic area in the supermarket is the household cleaning section. Children and expectant mothers must be protected from toxic environments.

The Canadian Partnership for Children's Health and Environment (CPCHE) recommends five actions to reduce common sources of toxic exposure associated with health risk, especially in children who are developmentally more vulnerable. These five recommendations are:

1. Control house dust.
2. Switch to less toxic, fragrance-free cleaners.
3. Take extreme care with renovation projects.
4. Avoid certain types and uses of plastics.
5. Eat fish that are low in mercury.

Today there are natural household products that can be made or purchased for the purposes of laundry, dish washing, dusting, bathroom and window cleaning, and more. Search the Web for natural cleaning products. Three common household items in your pantry can be used to clean most of your house: vinegar, lemon, and baking soda. Appendix C lists sources of natural cleaning products. You will be amazed at how simple healthy cleaning can be. Make it a weekly practice to open the windows (get a cross breeze if possible) to freshen the air in your home.

Atmosphere

Have you ever experienced being in a place and, for some reason, being there made you feel uncomfortable? Did you feel out of place and finally leave? It is important that our homes have the opposite effect by having a welcoming, peaceful, holistically clean environment. Use the Word of God to establish the overall foundation for living. You can declare the following mantras over your home:

❖ Put off thy shoes from thy feet: for the place where thou standest is holy ground. (Acts 7:33, KJV)

❖ Where the Spirit of the Lord is, there is liberty. (II Corinthians 3:17, KJV)

❖ As for me and my house, we will serve the Lord. (Joshua 24:15, KJV)

❖ Blessed is the man that walketh not in the counsel of the ungodly. (Psalm 1:1, KJV)

We must welcome the presence of the Trinity of God in our space. He is our provider, the protector of every threshold and chamber of our living space. We need to acknowledge His love and truth that provide the ability for each member and guest within this territory to be well and at peace. I have had many house guests who experienced noticeable improvements in their health as a result of being in our home. For instance, some guests with known food allergies, to their surprise, were able to eat those foods without an allergic reaction. One relative lived in our home for three months. When he arrived, he used 13 medications daily. By the end of the three-month period, he was down to three medications. All we did was go about our normal lifestyle of love, peace, and eating the purest of foods from whole grains, fruits, vegetables, and little-to-no animal products—and many of his chronic conditions went away!

As we move toward organizing our sacred spaces, our next step is to create boundaries. Each boundary serves as a healing chamber to help nurture the whole person. Boundaries help us designate areas for specific activities and habits of a wellness lifestyle. For example, smart phones, which serve as communication, information, and entertainment devices, can permeate every waking moment of our days if we are not careful. Soldiers on the battlefield for wellness cannot have a television in every room of the house. Knowing that television, the Internet, and radio are owned and operated outside the Kingdom of God, we cannot leave our minds open to these devices as constant background noise. Many of us fear silence, and yet silence invokes thought. For children of God, silence can pose great communion opportunities with the Father. In the silence of a moment, we can receive divine renewal and perspective.

In our sacred spaces, light and color play a significant role in creating a healing, nurturing environment. In Scripture, God said "Let there be light," (Genesis 1:3) and thus created color. Color has an impact on our trinity. Phyllis A. Balch, author of *Prescription for Nutritional Healing*, discusses color therapy in her book: "Color can be described as light—visible radiant energy—of certain wavelengths. Photoreceptors in the retina, called cones, translate this energy into colors." These cones work with the brain to perceive color. Balch also cites the research of Alexander Schauss, director of the American Institute for Biosocial Research, who concludes that the energy of color stimulates our pituitary and pineal glands. These glands impact the hormones that affect the physiological processes that influence our thoughts, moods, and behaviors. We can use color to help correct certain health issues and maintain our well-being.

Color	Common Effect	Use
Red	Energizes, heats, and promotes circulation. Causes strong feelings, increases physical energy, appetite, and can raise blood pressure. Also a sign of suffering, danger, and anger.	May be good during loss of appetite. Used in fast food establishments to encourage fast, large volume eating. Examples: Red sports cars, sexy red dress. May not be good for someone with high blood pressure; should not be used for those feeling anxious, angry, or with attention deficits.
Orange	Warms and cheers, frees bodily and emotional tension, mentally soothing. Promotes change as it is often seen in nature during the change of seasons. Stimulates vitamin C, known to promote lively conversations and great social events.	Shades of orange are a great color to use in kitchens and dining areas. Orange has a gentle warming effect if used lightly. Demands attention, but not like red does.
Yellow	A delightful color that lifts the spirit and encourages. Associated with the sun's life-giving rays, yellow can be used to help a person feel spiritually grounded and optimistic. Strengthens the nerves and aids self control and the intellect.	Notepads are typically yellow to stimulate thought and creativity. Great in kitchens and any room where happiness is needed.
Green	Color of life. It is the most restful color for the human eye. Associated with feeling grounded and calm. Promotes healing and relaxation. Refreshes. Stimulates growth; encourages healing of broken bones.	Use any shade to create a relaxing environment within your home. Used in hospitals and doctor's offices. Good font color in reading materials for seniors.
Blue	Helps restore a sense of inner peace and calm. Cooling and sedative. Helps ease pain and depression. Any shade connects with nature. Promotes truth and loyalty. Encourages good nutrition. Relaxes muscles. Reduces blood pressure & slows heart rate.	Perfect in rooms for rest. Use in bathrooms for a clean look and feel. Use in the kitchen to promote healthy digestion. Any ceiling in the home can be blue.
Violet	Associated with the imagination, strong faith, and the ability to use mind over matter. Brings balance and healing.	Use in rooms where calm and comfort are needed.

There are also certain values that complement our boundaries. Our values reflect the condition of our spirit and help us maintain that sense of peace. We have order which helps us thrive and move well. Consider the following items:

❖ **Leave shoes at the door.** Shoes are used for protection when away from home. The sacred home should not require this type of protection. All who enter should feel the peace and safety of this space. Environmentally, shoes contain toxins and dirt from everywhere (e.g., oil from cars, dirt, germs from a public restroom) and should not contaminate the inner areas of home.

❖ **Use no unnecessary chemicals.** In my home, we always ask, "Is there a natural alternative?"

❖ **Every word is a gift to the hearer** (Ephesians 4:29). Anger and emotions must be controlled and issues resolved. Be quick to hear, slow to speak, and slow to anger (James 1:19).

❖ To **avoid mindless eating,** there are only certain areas of the house where eating takes place.

❖ We need to **manage technology** and not allow technology to manage us. The Pew Research Center in a 2013 survey of 802 teenagers ages 12-17 and their parents reports that 78% of teens now have a cell phone, and almost half (47%) of those own smart phones, which provide seamless access to the Internet. One in four teens (23%) have a tablet computer and nine in ten (93%) teens have a computer or have access to one at home. It is important to do all things with moderation. Consider cut off points to technology. For example, shut down electronics one hour before bedtime and keep all charging stations to a common area. I conducted a survey of 150 teenagers and more than 60 percent of them slept with their cell phones under their pillow so they could engage in middle-of-the-night texting. House rules around technology are key.

❖ Strive for at least **one family meal per day.** This supports grounding and emotional health.

❖ **Silence is a gift.** Noise pollution does not promote wellness.

❖ Always **leave an area better** than you found it.

❖ **Respect the sacredness of sleep** and do not disturb others without real cause.

Healing Chambers

Kitchen and Bathrooms

Any real estate agent will tell you that the value of a home is significantly increased by the quality of the kitchen and bathrooms. I agree. Many people take that advice and remodel their homes, creating beautifully appealing rooms. Holistically speaking, the dollar value is an indirect benefit. The common sense part is that these two rooms set the stage for our health and well-being. Consciously or unconsciously, we know that these rooms are set apart: energy in, waste out. In the kitchen, the body is nourished with emotional and spiritual bonding taking place as we break bread and share with family and guests. The bathroom is where we cleanse ourselves from head to toe.

Therefore, it makes sense that these two rooms should be in good shape. They should reflect the love and values that subconsciously affect the peace and overall well-being of all who enter. These rooms should be neatly organized and maintained so that each family member is comfortable. The kitchen should be well lit, free of stale cooking odors and grease. Because colors influence us, never use red as a primary color in kitchen décor. Red increases heart rate and appetite. Red also causes us to eat quickly, something fast-food merchants have leveraged for years. The bathroom must be free of mold, mildew, dirt, and germs. The bathroom should also be brightly lit and cleaned with environmentally friendly cleaners. Shades of green and blue work well on the walls.

Bedrooms

> I laid me down and slept; I awaked; for the LORD sustained me.
> —Psalm 3:5 (KJV)

Our bedchambers are very important healing areas of our sacred space. We need a safe, clean, quiet place in which to have the mind, body, and spirit at rest.

Today there are so many activities going on in America's bedrooms. Poor sleep hygiene and sleep deprivation have become a public health issue.

According to a 2007 CDC survey from the Behavioral Risk Factor Surveillance System, 35.3 percent of adults reported less than seven hours of sleep in a typical 24-hour period. Seven to nine hours of sleep is recommended for adults. Over the years, I have observed from my clients that the bedroom has become a multiuse space. This is very common among children's bedrooms. We often create a little world for our kids. In this room, they have themed decorations of their favorite characters or sport. There are games and electronics, including computers and a desk for homework or crafts. It is a very busy place, and it can be difficult to get them to settle down to sleep. As adults, many of us bring everything into our bedrooms. The bedroom is an extension of what we do all day. When we eat in bed, talk on the phone in bed, watch television in bed, study for school or work on the laptop in bed, we send confusing messages to our bodies. The body tries to determine where it is located! "Am I still at school? Or am I in the kitchen?" Many people cap off the night by watching the evening news in bed. Overstimulation is common, making winding down very difficult. Sleep deprivation can be greatly reduced by the design, layout, and boundaries in the bedroom. Consider the following:

Situation	Explanation
There is no clutter.	Easier to clean; keeps the mind clear.
There are minimal electronics.	Creates sensory deprivation and reduces overstimulation. No television.
There is a comfortable chair for sitting and a nightstand to hold a glass of water and Bible or journal.	The chair is for sitting to prevent sitting on the bed.
The bed is used only for sleeping and legitimate intercourse.	The body has no mixed messages and is not violated.
Bedroom is a healing color.	Creates a calming, royal, natural environment.
There are several green plants.	Brings more oxygen and cleaner air.
There is as much natural light as possible with thick window coverings that can be moved when needed.	Bright and sunny by day. Allows for extended rest periods when needed.
There is a space designated as a prayer closet.	The place you go for your devotions, study, and prayer time with the Father.

Family Living Area

The home should also have a common area, where information sharing, recreation, and relaxation can occur. This area should be nurturing to every member of the household. It should also be a comfortable space for guests. Activities that take place can include studying God's Word during home Bible study, watching an occasional television program, playing board games, or listening to affirming, soothing music. This area should be functional based on family interests and age range of the household. Use colors that balance healing, warmth, and energy.

Organization

I have lived in many different spaces, including a tiny corner of a bedroom I shared with three sisters, a dorm room, an efficiency apartment, condominium, and multi-level homes. Keeping my space neat was helpful. As time went on, I realized that being organized was even better than being neat. In South Africa when I visited the villages, I noticed each home was very organized in the absence of what we in the United States would consider creature comforts. Even the one-room hut was organized. It was clear where the kitchen was versus the sleeping area. A space can be neat and look nice, but it may not be functional or set up to work based on your lifestyle and how you need to flow from day to day.

John Cherry, a minister and teacher on holistic living, stated in a presentation that, "Organization is God's key to simplify our lives." Imagine a Marine's barracks without a requirement or provision for organization: identical clothing and shoes all over the place, ammunition and weapons strewn about . . . you get the picture. Organization at home allows us to make the best of our territory. It frees the brain from the stress of navigating through stuff and allows us to move about freely, having an expectation on how to operate.

To support this expectation, I have added two additional rules to the John Cherry rule. The first is: **everything has a place.** We assign a place for an item and that is where we always expect it to be. This means no more looking for keys, cell phones, pencils, wallets, or socks! Everything has a place. The second rule is: **don't put it down and you will not have to pick it**

up. This is a powerful stress-relieving tool and a great time-saver. This rule also reinforces the idea that we handle things once. From mail to dirty socks, don't simply put them down, put them away.

With these rules, it is clear when our space is reaching inappropriate conditions. It allows us to control "stuff" and readily identify behaviors that threaten our peace and encourage reckless living. Controlling clutter is a good habit. Some experts suggest that it also supports mental clarity—all of which helps us stay well.

There is a correlation between our physical space and our mental capacity. Our thoughts can also be more organized. Journaling, as we discussed earlier in the prayer framework of Discipline 2, is an effective tool for clearing the mind. We can also connect the way we feel and what is important to us to the value system we spoke of earlier. We can see how we waste time and money on things and unhealthy relationships. There is a place for certain thoughts and feelings. We can see a relationship between such stressors as being late and being unable to perform tasks around the house. If I don't put a thought down right away (procrastination), then I will not have to face its potential consequences until another day.

Maintenance

A spirit of good communication and freedom, healing nature, and boundaries must be the norm, not the exception. A sacred space requires agreement from the head of the household and each family member to implement processes and accountability. A functional family of God requires prayer times, family meetings, roles and responsibilities for household chores, and timely home maintenance, including changing batteries in a smoke detector, collecting trash, and securing the house at night. Without these roles and responsibilities shared across all members of the household, a home can quickly become chaotic and affect everyone's health.

Finally, a sacred place requires discipline. It is an excellent training and development tool for children of all ages. It will help prepare them for sports, piano practice, or a job. It will help everyone in the home appreciate the sacredness of the space.

Sacred space in the workplace

Most of us spend a good portion of our day at work. Where possible, your space at work should reflect your values at home. There are some small things you can do to make work a healthier place.

Walk in peace. When you go to work, take peace—one of your spiritual weapons—along with you. Your workplace could harbor many stressors, including coworkers who are difficult to work with, environmental hazards, poor eating choices, or a micromanaging boss. Though you cannot control most of those external factors, you can control how you react to them; you can choose peace in the midst of mess.

Put together a work pantry. It could be a tin can or a few zip lock bags of healthy snacks. Your work pantry helps you maintain the power over your food intake. The vending machines should be avoided. Identify or bring a good source of water, and bring fresh fruit and vegetables everyday. Plan your lunch. If possible, pack your lunch.

Take breaks, which are vital to resting your body and mind. If your employer does not offer breaks, try to work with your boss or human resources representative to negotiate times when you can step away from your post to recharge. Reach towards home when you are on a break; check in with a loved one or friend by phone or e-mail if you can, or use the time to write and mail a card. A brief walk in the sunshine can work wonders for your body and rejuvenate your day.

Eating at your desk or while working is not recommended. It does not rest the mind or encourage life separate from work. It also is prone to cause more stress which often times leads to poor digestion.

Protect your body. If you sit most of the day, make sure you have a good chair and remember to stand and stretch. Multiple studies have shown that people who sit all day are more prone to heart disease than people who work on their feet. If you stand most of the day, invest in good, supportive shoes and a floor mat to help your legs. Use mouse pads with built-in wrist rests to prevent carpal tunnel.

Sacred space during travel

If you are one who is required to travel, you can create temporary living conditions that provide comfort and help maintain your wellness lifestyle. Here are a few tips:

- ❖ Once you reach your assigned space, be it a bunk bed at camp, hotel room, or suite:
    - o Declare that any evil or wrongdoing is arrested and cast out in Jesus' name. (Matthew 16:19)
    - o Welcome the spirit of God in, the Spirit of Peace, and His hedge of protection.
    - o Declare it to be holy ground fit for a child of Almighty God.
- ❖ Bring a small set of items from home, such as a towel or pillowcase to cover the pillow, a small picture of your family, and your favorite bar of soap, favorite snack, or tea bag.
- ❖ Research in advance where your best source of food is located. Search the Web for "health food." Include Asian (Chinese, Korean, Thai) and Indian cuisines in your search. If healthy options are not available, try to bring food from home.
- ❖ Travel with natural first aids:
    - o Aloe gel for cuts, burns, stings, and use as an astringent.
    - o Acidophilus/probiotic for diarrhea/food poisoning.
    - o Vitamin C for boosting the immune system.
    - o Arnica Montana gel and pellets for natural pain relief and anti-inflammation.

 Home should be different and more peaceful than any place outside.

 Home is my healing station, the place where I nurture wellness.

MOVE

> "You realize, don't you, that you are the temple of God, and God himself is present in you? No one will get by with vandalizing God's temple, you can be sure of that. God's temple is sacred—and you, remember, are the temple." —I Corinthians 3:16

L iving things move. A fit body is a body that moves. The body is the third part of the trinity of man. A soldier that remains fit has more capacity to live and serve in the Kingdom of God. She must not be weighed down. Being overweight and obese are associated with heart disease, cancer, type 2 diabetes, stroke, arthritis, breathing problems, and psychological disorders like depression. Lack of physical activity is one of the leading causes of chronic disease. A soldier is aware of the things that make him vulnerable. According to Christ, a good soldier must "stay alert. This is hazardous work I'm assigning you. You're going to be like sheep running through a wolf pack, so don't call attention to yourselves. Be as cunning as a snake, inoffensive as a dove" (Matthew 10:16).

Even when we are asleep, there is constant movement on the inside. Our bodies were given limbs, joints, sockets, and ligaments to allow movement without difficulty. No wellness lifestyle would be complete without some consistent exercise. We cannot be successful, however, unless we understand the real motivating factor to become and remain fit. It is not just for the sake of exercise and to have good-looking bodies. We move because it glorifies God. We are stewards of our bodies, not owners. Common sense tells us that our body is made for doing and moving, so we exercise the body to the glory of God.

The body was made to move. Our skeleton and joints were designed so that the body could move. In times past, there was enough movement built into daily living that an exercise program was not as important as it is today. Jesus was disciplined about exercise, as we see in several Scriptures. He walked from place to place and was a mountain climber. He and his disciples, many of whom were former commercial fishermen, were fit. His disciples had the ability to keep up with Jesus who went up and came down mountains.

We can work extra movement into our daily routine. For example when brushing my teeth, I do leg lifts (standing, holding on to the sink with the free hand). My husband often takes two steps at a time to stretch and push his body a little. A friend, when doing the laundry, does squats to pick up clothes. Another person, while sitting, rocks forward and backward to exercise the stomach muscles (like sit-ups). Others park their cars at the far end of the parking lot when shopping.

The fitness industry once had us convinced that exercise had to be formal training and rigorous, however, the Surgeon General and the American Heart Association have stated that walking can be of great benefit. Other activities include biking, dancing, jumping rope, swimming, running, tennis, basketball, sailing, hiking, skating, and more. It is important to remember that we must move every day and intensely three to four times a week for at least 30 minutes. Every day, I do a full body stretch, twist my waist, perform leg lifts, and try not to sit still for more than an hour without moving around. Four days out of the week, I repeat my daily routine and add a 2.5-mile uphill walk on the treadmill or in the park. This keeps me in enough shape to add many other activities, like dancing, taking the stairs, or hiking when possible.

Sedentary living is foolish behavior and not becoming of a soldier of Christ living in obedience for wellness. In a six-year study, Australian researchers discovered that people who said they watched television for more than four hours daily were 46 percent more likely to die of any cause and 80 percent more likely to die of heart disease than people who remain active. Even those who have jobs that require prolonged hours of sitting have an increased risk of heart disease. A sedentary lifestyle makes it far too easy to gain weight due to mindless eating and no activity.

As we age without movement and a proper diet, muscles waste away, balance lessens, flexibility deteriorates, heart and lung capacity decrease, posture (due to poor muscle mass and diet) worsens, and the spine curves. Discipline requires us to exercise and remain fit regardless of age. In the Bible, Caleb was one of the children of promise in Israel. As a young man, he was freed from Egyptian slavery. Years later in conversation with Joshua he said, "And here I am today, 85 years old! I'm as strong as I was the day Moses sent me out. I'm as strong as ever in battle, whether coming or going" (Joshua 14:11). As of this writing, my dad is 92 years old and still rollerblades. Dad has always moved beyond the normal activities of a day.

We exercise because we are soldiers whose bodies must be fit. Many people who are not overweight feel that a fitness routine is not necessary. A thin body does not mean good health. We were made to move. Movement tones our organs. The heart is a muscle and must be exercised beyond normal functions in order to remain strong. When fully expanded, our lungs exhale more stale air and help renew oxygen levels throughout the body. We cannot afford extra weight on our weight-bearing joints or to overwork our organs as they attempt to function with a blanket of fat around them.

Maintain Internal Body Functions

> Exercise pushes us beyond normal movements so that normal movements are easy.

Exercise pushes us beyond normal movements to ensure that normal movements are easy and injury-free. Regular exercise is a preventive measure that helps maintain internal body functions, such as:

- ❖ Boosting circulation and the flow of oxygen throughout the body
- ❖ Detoxifying the body through the sweat glands
- ❖ Regulating appetite and hormones
- ❖ Improving digestion and waste elimination
- ❖ Increasing energy levels
- ❖ Lowering cholesterol and blood pressure

❖ Reducing stress and anxiety

❖ Enhancing sleep

Movement is essential for proper core body functions. We develop flexibility by stretching. This relieves tension, relaxes the body, extends our reach, and aligns the spine. We should be able to touch every part of the body. A soldier should be able to lay hands and pray prayers of healing on any part of his body.

Cardio Fit – Healthy Heart

We increase heart capacity by increasing our heart rate through fast walking, running, biking, dancing, and various cardiovascular exercises. This gives us endurance. We should be able to take the stairs instead of the elevator anywhere. We should be able to act quickly in emergency situations. If you have a disability, consider what being in shape means for your situation. A physical therapist or trainer should be able to assist you with a fitness routine that works for you. For example, for a wheelchair-bound person, upper body strength is critical.

Fit Muscles

Building muscle mass and maintaining it is done by some degree of weight lifting or resistance exercises in which you use your own body. This allows us not to strain ourselves with groceries or any normal household task. Use muscles instead of your skeleton to hold your body erect when sitting or standing. Strong stomach muscles are important. Weak stomach muscles make for a weak back. See your stomach as a pot that needs a tight lid to hold it. Good posture is important for a fit body. Keep your spine straight by imagining a string from the ceiling attached to the top of your head pulling your shoulders and diaphragm up to the ceiling. Balance can be maintained by standing on one foot with arms stretched out on each side of your body, putting on socks, or washing feet without leaning on a wall.

Improve Breathing

Breathing exercises allow us to inhale good air, exhale bad air, and improve our lung capacity. See your lungs as two balloons. At least once a day breathe slowly and deeply to expand the balloons. Then exhale, pushing all the air out to flatten the balloons. This is a great exercise when we are doing our daily renewal prayer. It also helps reduce drowsiness. We should have the lung capacity to run for short distances or walk very fast.

Moving During the Winter Months

A fitness routine for the winter months can be more difficult. The long, cold nights make it easy to become demotivated and exclude exercise from our adjusted schedules caused by shorter days. It will be important to plan for this change so that we have a seamless transition into the next season. Because the winter months are also filled with many holiday socials (eating, eating, and more eating) with a more demanding schedule, it will be easy to put fitness on hold in order to meet other commitments. This time of year also tests our ability to maintain the Seven Disciplines. Consider jumping rope, hula hooping, or mall walking. (Search the Web for "mall walkers association.") I have a pair of 2 pound dumbbells. Some days I turn on my favorite upbeat gospel music and start moving. I use gospel music because it serves two purposes: a praise opportunity and a workout. You could add more reps to climbing the stairs at work or at home, join the Y or gym, or get a buddy or prayer partner to walk with you.

Motivation to Keep Moving

One of the easiest ways to make exercise a part of your lifestyle is to resolve in your **mind** that living things move. And like David, **choose** to live—not die—to the glory of God, the giver of life (Psalm 118:17). Sitting around and eating more food than the body can use causes the body to hold on to extra fat and, over time, makes us weak. A lifestyle on God's terms includes remembering that we are temples of the Holy Spirit in a battle to complete our assignment. There is a relationship between our walk with Christ and how we treat our bodies. We must repent of any abuse to our bodies. "As ye have therefore received Christ Jesus the Lord, so *walk* ye in him" (Colossians 2:6, KJV). With forgiveness and a renewed mind, ask your loving Father God to help you with the exercise routine that works for you. Adjust for the seasons. And do it! Call your doctor and let him know.

Exercise engages the entire trinity in order to become disciplined about moving the body. No soldier can fight without movement. No runner can win a race unless she moves. Being able to fit into a size eight dress or that favorite sports jacket is not the motivation for exercising. When we move our bodies to be fit, we reflect the healthy condition of our trinity, not just the body. We move because we love God and appreciate the property He has entrusted to us. The Apostle Paul put it this way: "I don't know about you, but I'm running hard for the finish line. I'm giving it everything I've got. No sloppy living for me! I'm staying alert and in top condition. I'm not going to get caught napping" (I Corinthians 9:26-27).

> A wise man is strong; yea, a man of knowledge increaseth strength.
> —Proverbs 24:5 (KJV)

 Everything that lives moves.

 The Holy Spirit moves, my body moves also.

EAT AND DRINK REAL FOOD

I n the diseased culture, wellness is primarily based on how we eat. It is a billion-dollar industry with a new expert born every day, presenting the latest diet and eating regimen. Because wellness is so much more than food, I decided to make it the last discipline. Like moving, eating for appearance is not sustainable. For soldiers in Christ's army, eating and drinking is an issue of stewardship.

We have discussed the spiritual nourishment needed to promote spiritual health that is connected to God through Jesus Christ. We also discussed the emotional and mental food requirements that come from our knowledge, obedience to the instructions for living outlined in the Word of God, our prayer life, and thought life. Now we need to discuss the significance of a good diet for our temple, which undergirds the ability for complete trinity wellness. As a soldier in Christ's army, we must stand guard to ensure that the food we eat is strengthening for our journey and not a tool of the enemy to weaken us and undermine our health.

Historically, as the world population grew, more food sources were required. According to some historical facts, 300 years ago only 600 million people needed to be fed. Today, industrialized agriculture attempts to feed 7 billion people. War and industry offered alternative employment instead of farming. Demand increased for farmers to grow more and transport food to regions where people lived but no longer farmed. Industrialized farming replaced growing your own food.

We have gone from gathering our own food for meals to having an industrial complex deliver food by way of greenhouses, warehouses, trucks, and ships. In the U.S., we produce over 3,000 calories per day for each citizen. Our fruits and vegetables are harvested under-ripened, and thus less nutritious, so they can get to market prior to perishing. Some are genetically modified organisms (GMOs), meaning a scientist intervenes to change the properties of a plant. Many see this as harmless. But it is a fact that many of our fruit like grapes, oranges, and melons can no longer reproduce themselves as God intended because they are genetically modified to lack seeds. Most of the corn grown in the United States is from a seed that contains a pesticide that deters insects and worms. There are companies today that are rapidly acquiring patents on seeds that will prevent use of those seeds without permission. This means a few people, not nature, may control the ongoing availability of certain crops. Animals are raised indoors and are rarely exposed to sunlight or allowed to move about freely. They are constantly medicated in order to keep them from getting sick. Cows are fed corn instead of grass. This corn diet overrides the grass diet innate to cows and causes a digestive nightmare for these creatures. Animal growth hormones are used to speed up the arrival time to market and increase volume. We no longer have relationships with the food we consume. When food is prepared for an extended shelf life, we lose nutrients and our connectedness to our food.

While we were not being watchful, the food supply has changed. **Everything that is being called food is not necessarily real food.** There are many nonfood items in food. When we ingest nonfood items, the body has to address them, without benefit and often losing strength as a result. Michael Van Straten, author of *The Healthy Food Directory* states, "High-fat, high-salt, high-sugar products, storage processing, intensive farming, growth hormones and antibiotics have not added to the nutritional value of what we eat today." Food additives are approved by the Food and Drug Administration (FDA), for "safety" and can be added to our food. These additives include dyes, stabilizers, preservatives, and taste enhancers.

There are more than 3,000 total substances that comprise an inventory referred to as *Everything Added to Food in the United States* (EAFUS). The EAFUS list of substances contains ingredients added directly to food that the FDA has either approved as food additives or listed or affirmed as Generally Recognized As Safe (GRAS). When we read food labels, most of these ingredients have long chemical terms. Some of these items have no known risks; however some of them are proven dangerous in animals. We must also consider our individual health conditions. While these nonfoods are recognized as safe, no one knows the synergistic effect of these chemicals being ingested simultaneously. We don't always know how our body responds to these chemicals when we use them while taking prescription medicines or over-the-counter pain relievers.

There are also harmful pesticides being used on our nation's produce, which should be avoided. The increased availability of organic foods has been helpful, but the cost makes them unaffordable for the average household. **Organic foods** are grains, produce, and meats that have been raised without the use of harmful chemicals, pesticides, or pharmaceuticals. This category of food must comply with rigorous agricultural standards. Foods that are locally grown or are grown within the region where you live may not be organic, but they will normally have fewer chemicals because of the short distance to market. If organic or local produce are not options, fresh vegetables are still better than no vegetables. To remove a great deal of the pesticides, wax, and other residue, use a vegetable wash or add ½ cup of apple cider vinegar, or five drops of grapefruit seed extract, to approximately one gallon of water. Soak the produce for 10 minutes, then rinse well.

The Environmental Working Group, a nonprofit environmental research group helps us prioritize our organic purchases by identifying the produce that contains the highest pesticide residues. The following is a list of foods that have little to no pesticide residues and are considered safe to purchase without being organic: **asparagus, avocado, banana, broccoli, cabbage, kiwi, mango, onion, papaya, pineapple, sweet corn (frozen), sweet peas (frozen).**

The following foods are conventionally grown with high amounts of pesticides. Consumers are therefore cautioned to buy certified organic versions of these foods, which are grown with fewer or no pesticides: **apple, celery, cherry, grape (imported), lettuce, nectarine, peach, pear, potato, strawberry, spinach, sweet bell pepper.**

As Satan would have it, many foods have been denatured by processing to the point that their nutritional value has been depleted. For example, raw milk was at one time considered a therapeutic agent for restoring the health and strength of the sick. Due to processing and necessary safety requirements, however, raw milk is illegal in most states. When milk is heated (pasteurized then homogenized), the medicinal properties are destroyed. Bread is another example of food that was clearly intended to keep the body strong. However, the grains used to make bread today have been stripped of the nutrient-dense outer layer, and as a result most of the nutrients are lost.

God's Original Diet

> And God said, Behold, I have given you every herb bearing seed, which is upon the face of all the earth, and every tree, in the which is the fruit of a tree yielding seed; to you it shall be for meat.
> —Genesis 1:29 (KJV)

If we look in Genesis 1:27-29, we see that man was created from the dirt. God immediately gave the first couple a tour of the garden to show them how to feed themselves. He presented all types of plants, herbs, fruits, and vegetables to be eaten as "meat." God's intention was that the body would be sustained by eating the plants He had provided. The blood of green plants, chlorophyll, is almost identical to our blood. Common sense should tell us that a plant-based diet is critical to the health and strength of the body. Food is to be our medicine.

God allowed the children of Israel to eat the flesh of certain animals and fish (Deuteronomy 14:4-21). He never said that these items were replacements for plants. They are additions, not substitutes for plants, and should be eaten occasionally.

Scripture also makes it clear that we should avoid those foods that deceive us by tasting good but lacking the nutrients needed to heal and prevent diseases.

The significance of a plant-based diet has been scientifically proven as well. One such study is The China Study conducted by Dr. T. Colin Campbell, who outlines the connection between nutrition and heart disease, diabetes, and cancer, and nutrition's ability to reduce or reverse the effects of these deadly illnesses. This 20-year study proved that "people who ate the most animal-based foods got the most chronic disease. . . People who ate the most plant-based foods were the healthiest and tended to avoid chronic disease."

> When you sit down to eat with a ruler, consider carefully what is before you; and put a knife to your throat if you are a man given to appetite. Do not desire his delicacies, for they are **deceptive food**.
> —Proverbs 23:1-3 (NKJV)

God made the body from the earth. We must feed it those foods that are directly from the earth. Our cells are programmed to expect the best of nutrients, which reproduce, detoxify, and sustain the body. The body is programmed to expect and effectively use the foods contained in the original diet to keep itself healthy.

All plants, including fruits, vegetables, and grains, receive energy from the sun and from nutrient-rich soil. The energy and nutrients are then transferred to us as we eat them. Food is electricity for our bodies. Foods eaten in their original state, or unprocessed, are healthier. For example, it is better to eat an apple instead of having applesauce or apple juice that has been heated and processed. The raw apple provides nutrients and fiber from its skin. Juice is more concentrated, has more sugar, and is often pasteurized. Applesauce is cooked, provides less fiber, with possible additives and preservatives. The fibrous portions of plants and fruits are not digested. God's self-healing strategy is that fiber scrubs the digestive tract to prevent buildup and inflammation within our waste channels. Whole grains are foundational for a healthy diet. In Scripture, when God ministered to the children of Israel, He instructed them to use grains to build strength. "Also take for yourself wheat, barley, beans, lentils, millet, and spelt; put them in one vessel, and make bread of them for yourself" (Ezekiel 4:9, NKJV). In II Samuel 17, David and his people were given wheat, barley, flour, parched grain, beans, lentils, and parched seeds to strengthen and encourage them in the wilderness. Grains are the best source of protein because they regulate blood sugar and provide a rich source of vitamins and minerals.

So why didn't Christ choose fish and chips or a leg of lamb for the last supper (I Corinthians 11:23-26)? He used symbols that sustain our trinity. He chose whole grain bread for its life-strengthening properties to represent his body, and wine (grapes) that contains resveratrol, a powerful antioxidant (cleanser) and protector of brain tissue, to represent his blood. Christ gave us life and cleansed our blood. We went from having Adam's blood contaminated with sin to being infused with the uncontaminated blood of Christ, the second Adam.

The Challenge with Eating Right

The typical American diet is a blessing and a curse. It is a blessing that we have such a large variety of foods that are reasonably priced, easy to prepare, and taste good. It is a curse, however, for almost the same reasons, in addition to the fact that God's children must refrain from those foods that weaken the body. Our convenient access to a variety of foods makes it easy to choose foods that taste good, not necessarily those that the body needs to be strong. Many foods that are most convenient do not provide the nutritional components the body needs to maintain good health. Dr. Terry Dorian, author of *Health Begins in Him* writes, "If we are disciplined and enlightened consumers, we will have no need for the majority of food products offered in American supermarkets." Dorian continues, "These are foods which are first devitalized and then filled with chemicals, flavorings, hydrogenated oils, sugar, artificial sweeteners, and dyes." These are the deceptive foods we are told to avoid in Proverbs 23:1-3.

Being in the world but not of the world means being within the Kingdom of God. This should be a constant reminder that our lifestyle is sustainable based on the love and knowledge of our Father God. The food supply in the world is one that is led by those who agree consciously or unconsciously to the production of food that supports disease and death. These foods contain large amounts of bad fat, sugar, and sodium, which drain energy and increase the risk of heart disease, cancer, high blood pressure, diabetes, and obesity. The enemy has again taken what God created to sustain us and changed the truth. For example, the bread that is to strengthen us according to Ezekiel 4:9 is not the bread most available today. Bread today has been stripped of the nutritional layers, bleached white, sweetened, and preserved. Yet we still consume large amounts of it and it is a major contributing factor of diabetes.

The blending of cultures in the U.S. and the marketing of the most profitable morsels have made us very vulnerable to the buzz and glitter of packages containing the latest food fads and diets. When we fail to use common sense about our food, it is easy to forget that food is energy. "When we consume these foods, we damage our bodies at the cellular level," Dorian states. In loving ourselves, we must pursue the best quality energy that we can. Surveys have shown that less than 22 percent of high school students and only 24 percent of adults reported eating the recommended five or more servings of fruits and vegetables per day.

The teaching of Hippocrates reinforces God's plan for healing the body and still rings true today: "Let your food be your medicine and your medicine be your food."

Real food comes directly from the garden and the farm. Real food should remain close to its original state when we consume it. God made us from dirt; we should consume foods from dirt. We are kin to these foods. Chlorophyll from vegetables is almost identical to human hemoglobin, which makes it an almost-perfect food for restoring, cleansing, and strengthening the body. The best meals are those that remain intact when we prepare them.

When it comes to being well and eating meat and sugar, less is best. These are part of the deceptive foods referred to in Proverbs 23:1-3. The kings and rulers of that day were rich and powerful. They indulged in costly foods that were prepared for taste. These foods weakened the body. In the Book of Daniel (Daniel 1:15-16), we read how Daniel and three other Hebrew men were vegetarians when the Babylonians captured them. They were given choice foods from the king's table. These men rejected the king's food and proved that their way of eating made their bodies stronger than those men who ate from the king's table.

In Scripture, eating animal meat was added to the diet, however, it was never said to be a replacement for grains, vegetables, and fruit outlined in the original diet. Americans consume three times more meat than the global average, which greatly impacts our ability to prevent chronic disease, according to the National Cancer Institute. It is clear that a plant-based diet was what God intended, which Scripture refers to as meat (I Kings 19:8; Genesis 1:29-30; Leviticus 2:1,4).

God distinctively said in Leviticus that blood was not to be eaten. "Life is in the blood" according to Leviticus 17:14. Dr. M.R. DeHaan in his book *The Chemistry of the Blood* discusses the New and Old Testament edict from God that we should not eat blood or anything that contains blood, such as meat (Genesis 9:4, Leviticus 7:26-27, Acts 15:28-29). This is why kosher meats are drained and soaked in salted water: to remove all blood from the animals prior to eating. When I was a child, I remember seeing my mother soaking her meats and chicken in large bowls of salted water, never really making the connection before now. The diseased culture has flipped the truth. We fry fat and eat it, which was also forbidden (Leviticus 7:23). Fat clogs the arteries of the heart and raises blood pressure. Meat has become a staple and a sign of wealth—the bloodier, the better. If meat from animals is not present on the plate or menu, it is seen as a poor quality meal, creating a sense of depravity and hence not a very good eating experience. Many see vegetables as oversized garnishes that are optional. When grains are eaten, most people prefer them white and buttery.

The truth is that every nutrient we need is within plants. Even protein and calcium, two nutrients most people think cannot be obtained without an animal source, are found within plants. A diet that consists of primarily meat and white foods, including rice, bread, and pasta, are deceptive foods that do not provide the essential nutrients or fiber needed to keep the body from sickness and disease. The healthiest people in the world, according to The China Study, have a plant-based diet.

Many followers of Christ feel that the New Testament reverses the dietary plan that was laid out in the Old Testament. Not so; **the body has not changed.** One such Scripture is the letter from the Apostle Paul to the Roman Christians reminding them to be peacemakers and followers of Christ first. He also reminds us that God has invited everyone to come to Christ's table regardless of background or lifestyle (Romans 14:2-3). Paul asked them not to be disruptive to the eaters of meat or the vegetarians. All food is good but will turn bad if you use it badly (Romans 14:20-21). So, come as you are. As more truth is revealed and we mature in the freedom of Christ, we will grow into healthier eating habits.

I am also convinced that food in and of itself will not keep you well. What keeps us well is our desire to live on God's terms. We do His will through our obedience to His Word and the personal, unique relationship we have with Him through Jesus and the Holy Spirit in us. God outlines in His Word a disciplined way and foods that correspond with the way He made the human body, which is self-healing. When Paul said all food is good, I agree. In the absence of common sense, however, **we have been led to believe that all that is called "food" today is the same food God provided. It is not.**

Today's food is contaminated by the diseased culture with genetically modified organisms, artificial flavors, unnatural preservatives, hormones, pesticides, herbicides, and waxes. Our food supply has become a warehouse of untruths masterminded by Satan to bring God's creation to a state of weakness and early destruction. As a result, we are tired and so sick—in mind and body. Our spirits are broken and discouraged and we live unsuspecting the relationship between what we eat and how we feel and think. Food has energy; we take on the attributes of whatever we eat. As with the flesh-eating lion that is aggressive and unpredictable, so is the easygoing vegetarian elephant or giraffe. When we eat bloody meat, we take on the temperament and medical history of that animal. It does not appear that God would have us ingest the DNA of lower animals to keep our bodies strong and well. Whenever we are enslaved without choice, God our provider will bless whatever we have to eat as long as we have a grateful heart.

Where to Start?

The enemy has used food for a long time to separate us from God. Today the fight has become more difficult and clever. This means we have to be watchful and selective about what we eat. Getting some advice from a friend who has lost 20 pounds is great, however, we will need our God to assist us. We will need to use the weapons He has provided to move us toward those foods that allow us to have strength within His Kingdom.

> That triggered a response from one of the guests: "How fortunate the one who gets to eat dinner in God's kingdom!" —Luke 14:15

To get started, we have to change the way we think about food. If we go along with the crowd and eat whatever is presented, we will become weak. Food is mainly for energy and healing. A helpful prayer that I give to my clients and students is "Lord, please change my palate to desire those foods that make me well." The meal setting or environment might change, be it a party or celebration with family and friends. We should avoid mindless eating, which often happens while watching television or a movie or while we are bored. When we eat for anything other than nourishment to keep the body strong, food becomes a dangerous, multiuse item. When food is before you, ask the questions: "Am I eating for energy and healing or for another reason? What is the nutrient value of this food, and does my body need it? Is it too close to bedtime to eat this?" Using the answers to these questions, the disciplined soldier will recognize the risks and will be able to pass on the hot wings or to eat very little to none of that birthday cake!

We must ask God to change our taste buds to desire those foods that are pure and life-giving. In time, as we use the truth about food, we will begin to recognize real food. You will have the intelligence and self-control of a soldier to resist the magnetic pull of food traps. Like seedless fruit that cannot reproduce themselves, many of our foods do not provide the nutrients we need to produce the next generation of healthy cells to keep us well and productive.

A Soldier's Diet

The body requires some basic nutrients every day. I have listed the nutrient and the best to worst sources of these nutrients. The worst sources are those that are very common in the American diet. Other than lack of physical fitness, these foods are the leading causes of chronic disease.

> Give us this day our daily bread. —Matthew 6:11 (KJV)

Transitioning to God's Original Diet

If you know that you currently are not eating and drinking real food, then reading this chapter and moving forward might seem overwhelming. The following steps can help you slowly transition into healthier eating practices:

1. **Pray about it.** Ask the Father to forgive you for the careless eating of your past, and ask Him to change you taste buds to desire those foods that make and keep you well.

2. Use the **"once in a while" concept.** As you transition to eating healthy, it is important not to totally cut out all of your favorite foods in the first week. Doing so can trigger symptoms of withdrawal and depression that can prevent you from moving forward. It's important to wean yourself off of unhealthy foods slowly so your body and mind have time to adapt. Consider what you eat currently and replace it with God's original way of eating. Then, *once in a while*, eat something that you eat now, even if it is unhealthy. In the beginning, eat your "once in a while" meal once a week. Then after a few weeks, eat your "once in a while" meal every other week. Then eat it only once a month. After a few months of weaning yourself off the unhealthy food, your taste buds will be less willing to eat those less nourishing foods. By the end, your body should only crave a slice of Aunt Margaret's pie on Thanksgiving. Remember this: it is not what you eat once in a while. It is what you eat everyday that counts.

3. **Convert your pantry.** Consider every item in your pantry (refrigerator and cabinets). As you run out of something, replace it with something healthier. For example, replace the refined wheat crackers with whole grain crackers that are lower is sodium and preservatives and loaded with fiber and nutrients. When the cow's milk runs out, replace it with one of the plant milks like almond, soy or rice milk, which are naturally free of cholesterol and bad fats.

Basic Nutrients for a Healthy Diet

Our need for food was intentional by God to sustain us and help us enjoy constant communion with Him for as long as we live. We have developed a practice of giving thanks to God for our food at the table just prior to eating. A soldier must be prayerful during the selection, gathering, and preparation of food. The Holy Spirit within you will assist you with what you should have for each meal each day that you live.

Protein	**Best sources:** Beans, peas, nuts, seeds, vegetables, potatoes, whole grains, fish
	OK sources: Poultry, small amounts of red meat, eggs, dairy
	Worst sources: Fried chicken, fried seafood, pizzas, burgers, whole milk, butter, cheese, red meat, pork, shellfish
	Note: The American Dietetic Association has stated that adequate protein can be obtained without meat (July 1, 2009). www.eatright.org
Carbohydrates	**Best sources:** Fresh fruit and vegetables, whole grains
	Worst sources: Refined sugar, candy, white flour/pasta, baked goods, and white grains
Fats	**Best sources:** Oils: olive, canola, safflower, sesame, and unheated flaxseed, fish oil
	Worst sources: Vegetable oil. Saturated fats from meat, dairy, margarines, shortenings, and products using these ingredients.

For a long time, the enemy has used food, both physical and spiritual, to separate us from God. Today the fight has become more difficult and clever. This means we must be watchful and selective about what we eat, applying the common sense truth of the Word of God.

Think of missionaries. When they travel to foreign lands, they cannot eat most of what the native population eats, because their bodies are not used to the contamination that exists within the native food and water. They must search for food, eat only what they need, and try to plan for several future meals. We are near to a food famine. Pure food is difficult to find, costly, and nonexistent in some parts of the country. These "nutritional deserts" have only deceptive foods. There are no fresh foods and no suppliers within certain communities. As a result, disease is increasing, and nutritional deprivation is affecting younger populations and their children.

Now that we know what deceptive foods are, we must put aside everything that would prevent us from accomplishing the work the Father has assigned to us. We know that too much meat, oil, sugar, and grains stripped of nutrients will destroy God's temples (our bodies).

In order to remain strong, we must embrace the diet designed for a child of God. Common sense based on Scripture makes the following statements clear:

❖ We need to have a plant-based diet.

❖ Less is best.

❖ Pure is sure.

❖ Honoring God is what motivates us to eat well.

We Need a Plant-Based Diet

The plate for a plant-based diet should contain more food from a plant origin and little from animal protein and fish (not shellfish). Scripture places a clear emphasis on eating grains. The original diet is based on plant eating and is referred to as "meat." In I Kings 19:5-8, we see that God's provision for the prophet Elijah was bread, which God called "meat." This meat was to sustain Elijah for 40 days. This speaks to the power and quality of nutrients supplied to us through grains. A healthy plate can be achieved without animal protein using whole grains, beans, nuts, seeds, and vegetables.

Plate for a Plant-Based Diet

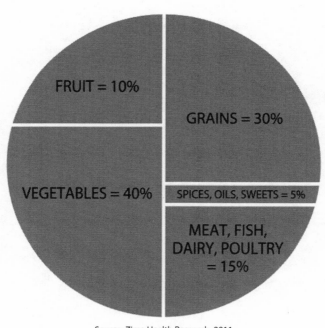

Source: Zima Health Research, 2011

Food	Nutrient Features	Common Sources
Vegetables	Vitamins, minerals, chlorophyll, and protein. Note: This information is helpful for regulating blood sugar.	**Non-starchy:** Cucumber, broccoli, cauliflower, celery, turnip, radish, onion, green bean, sweet corn, sweet pea, zucchini, leek, garlic, eggplant, bell pepper, mushroom, asparagus, summer squash, okra, chard, kale, spinach, parsley, watercress, lettuce, cabbage, bok choy, mustard, collard and beet greens, sprouts of alfalfa, seaweed and micro-algae (spirulina, wild blue-green, chlorella) **Starchy:** Potato, sweet potato, beet, parsnip, carrot, pumpkin, winter squash
Fruit	Carbohydrates; excellent source of vitamins, minerals. Fruit can be divided into four categories: acid, sub-acid, sweet and melons. For optimal digestion it is best not to mix types. For example, eat any combination of melons at the same time, but don't eat grapes, oranges or apples at the same time as melons.	**Acid:** Orange, lemon, grapefruit lime, pineapple, tangelo, pomegranate, tangerine, strawberry, cranberry **Sub-Acid:** Peach, berries, pear, apple, mango, apricot, papaya, plum **Sweet:** Banana, persimmon, grape, mango, papaya, cherry, fig, sapodilla, dried fruits **Melons:** Watermelon, crenshaw, muskmelon, cantaloupe, charentais, Persian casaba, honeydew
Whole grains	Whole grains are unprocessed and contain protein, carbohydrates, oil, vitamins, minerals, and bran.	Whole unrefined cereals, breads and pasta including wheat, quinoa, millet, rice, rye, barley, buckwheat, spelt, corn, oats, kamut, amaranth
Meat and dairy	Protein, vitamins B_6 and B_{12}, zinc, selenium, and fatty acids.	Red meat: beef, lamb, pork Poultry: chicken, duck, goose, turkey, game, eggs Dairy: milk, cheese, butter
Seafood	Protein, B vitamins, iron, and zinc. Oily fish contain vitamin D, omega-3 fatty acids and calcium.	Fish with fins, shellfish.
Legumes	Beans, peas, lentils. High in protein, fat, and carbohydrates. Rich in potassium, calcium, iron, and several B vitamins.	Aduki beans, black beans, lentils, green split peas, whole peas, kidney beans, garbanzo beans, lima beans, black-eyed peas, mung beans, soy beans
Nuts and seeds	Rich source of protein, fat, many minerals, some fiber, and B-complex vitamins.	Almonds, black sesame seeds, Brazil nuts, cashews, chia seeds, coconut, flax seeds, peanuts, pine nuts, pecans, pistachios, pumpkin, and squash seeds, sunflower seeds, walnuts
Oils	Good fats	Flax seed, extra virgin olive oil, unrefined sesame oil, canola and safflower oils, fish, nuts, seeds, avocados.

Vegetables and fruits are important for optimal weight management and chronic disease prevention. *The Dietary Guidelines for Americans* recommend 2 to 6½ cups of fruits and vegetables (four to 13 servings) per day. God provided fruit, vegetables, and grains as the healing agents to detoxify, restore, and heal our bodies. Fresh fruit should be consumed as opposed to processed fruit in sugar-sweetened syrup. We should eat whole vegetables or fruit in place of juices. Vegetables can be raw, lightly steamed, stir-fried, roasted, or added to soups. Eat fresh, frozen, or canned vegetables without high-calorie sauces and added salt.

Vegetables fresh from the farm or just picked are more nutritious than their frozen or canned counterparts. But frozen and canned vegetables are an acceptable nutritional alternative, according to the nation's dietary guidelines and the National Institute of Health. Consideration must still be given for the amount of salt added to canned vegetables, which could be harmful. However, common sense should tell us that the time from harvest to table impacts the nutritional value of our food. These are the types of fruits and vegetables, **in order of priority**, I recommend to maximize the quality of every nutrient:

- ❖ Certified organic
- ❖ Locally grown
- ❖ Conventional
- ❖ Frozen
- ❖ Low-sodium, canned

Grains should include more whole grain cereals, brown rice, whole grain pasta, corn, whole grain couscous, quinoa, barley, and less wheat products. Over-consumption of wheat has caused an increase in allergies. Whole grains help regulate blood sugar at an optimum level for longer periods as they are slowly absorbed into the body.

Meat, including poultry, should be consumed less. Meat and shellfish are the major sources of dietary cholesterol. The body naturally produces cholesterol and is not in need of another source. Therefore, meatless meals at least twice or more a week are highly recommended. Limit processed meats that are high in saturated fat and sodium. Less is best, which prevents gluttonous behaviors. Meat should be baked, roasted, or gas-grilled, not fried. Use lean cuts of meat and remove skin from poultry before eating. The American Heart Association recommends fish twice a week, preferably oily fish including salmon, mackerel, or tuna. The cholesterol content of shellfish is very high and is not recommended. Avoiding shrimp, crab, or lobster corresponds to the biblical instructions to eat only fish with fins and scales (Deuteronomy 14:10).

Many populations in various parts of the world do not use dairy products as a part of their diet. Their calcium intake is from plant sources. In our country, calcium deficiencies are prevalent, which puts many people at risk of arthritis and osteoporosis.

A common myth about calcium is that dairy is the best source. There are many sources of calcium from plant-based sources. Appendix D lists those sources. Excessive meat consumption has been linked to calcium deficiency, according to Paul Pitchford in his book *Healing with Whole Foods*. Pitchford also adds that our bodies often do not absorb calcium due to other foods and substances ingested.

Calcium Absorption Inhibitors

- ❖ Coffee, soft drinks, and diuretics
- ❖ Excesses of protein, especially meat
- ❖ Refined sugar or too much concentrated sweetener
- ❖ Alcohol, marijuana, cigarettes, and other intoxicants
- ❖ Too little or too much exercise
- ❖ Excess salt
- ❖ Nightshades: tomatoes, potatoes, eggplant, and bell peppers
- ❖ Lack of magnesium, which is needed for bone health

Beans, peas, and legumes are excellent plant protein sources. When consumed with grains or vegetables, we are able to provide our bodies all of the nutrients required for a healthy meal without meat.

Oils (fats) are an essential nutrient of the body. Many of us have come to believe that we do not need fat and that fat is bad. The type of fat we need, however, has been replaced by inferior sources that make the body weak and diseased. The fat-free industry has introduced products that contain non-food chemical concoctions that are not detected as fat and pass through the system. The truth is that every cell in the body needs fat. The wall of each cell is fat, which should indicate that fat is pretty important. The following are the good and bad fats currently in our food supply.

Good Fats	
Monounsaturated fat	Olive oil, peanut oil, canola oil, avocados, nuts, seeds
Polyunsaturated fat	Vegetable oils (such as safflower, corn, sunflower, soy, and cottonseed), nuts, seeds
Omega-3 fatty acids	Fatty, cold-water fish (such as salmon, mackerel, and herring), fish oil, flax seeds, flax oil, walnuts

Bad Fats (Avoid)	
Saturated fat	Animal products (meat, poultry, seafood, eggs, dairy products, lard, butter), coconut, palm, and other tropical oils
Trans fat	Partially hydrogenated vegetable oils, margarine, shortening, commercially baked goods (crackers, cookies, cakes), fried foods (doughnuts, French fries)
Dietary cholesterol	Animal products (meat, poultry, seafood, eggs, dairy products, lard, butter)

Less is Best

Earlier we stated that the food industry produces about 3,000 calories per day for each American. This is an average of 700 more calories than should be consumed based on gender and age. Obesity during biblical times was a sign of wealth. The rich people could lie around and indulge in expensive, high fat, sugary diets. Today it is just the opposite.

It is best for a soldier to remain fit by eating less. Scripture warns us about overeating:

> Do not associate with winebibbers; be not among them nor among
> gluttonous eaters of meat, for the drunkard and the glutton shall come
> to poverty. (Proverbs 23:20-21, AMP)

Food eaten in excess is intoxicating and sedative. It puts the digestive system at capacity, pulls energy, and slows down activity in order to address the massive amount of calories consumed. We are also warned not to have a full stomach, which may prevent good sleep (Ecclesiastes 5:12).

When we eat, the body uses what it needs for fuel and whatever is not needed spills over into storage areas of the body to be used at another time. Because we habitually consume the same amount of calories, the body never has a demand to use the energy from storage.

It is not good to eat much honey. —Proverbs 25:27 (KJV)

According to the Nutrition Division of the CDC, too much protein from animal sources can be harmful. Animal proteins are the major sources of saturated fat which has been linked to elevated low-density lipoprotein (LDL) cholesterol, a risk factor for heart disease. In addition, for people with certain kidney diseases, a lower-protein diet is recommended to help prevent weak kidney function, according to Mayo Clinic nutritionists.

Too many refined carbohydrates can be harmful to the body. These refined carbohydrates include refined sugar and grains that have been stripped of the outer layers of the grain (the bran and the germ). When these two layers are removed during the milling process, we lose key essential vitamins and minerals like selenium and magnesium.

Avoid sugar with the awareness that it has been added to almost every item in our nation's food supply. From toothpaste to bread, sugar is there. The American Heart Association recommends limiting sugar sweetened beverages to less than 450 calories per week (36 ounces). The *Dietary Guidelines for Americans 2010* indicates the healthiest way to reduce caloric intake is to decrease consumption of added sugars, which provide calories but few or no essential nutrients. The names of sugars include:

Brown sugar	High-fructose corn syrup	Molasses
Corn sweetener	Honey	Raw sugar
Corn syrup	Invert sugar	Sucrose
Dextrose	Lactose	Sugar
Fruit juice concentrate	Maltose	Syrup corn
Glucose	Malt syrup	

Sugars that are **safe in moderate use** include rice syrup, barley malt, date sugar, stevia, agave nectar, and maple syrup.

Avoiding sodium is also difficult. It is estimated that the average American ingests more than 3,000 mg of sodium per day, which is twice the recommended amount. Sodium intake should be 1,500 mg or less per day. Here are some suggestions to help:

❖ Choose and prepare foods with little or no salt.

❖ Limit the use of condiments such as soy sauce and ketchup.

❖ If choosing processed foods, look for the lowest in sodium.

❖ Compare the sodium content of various brands and choose those with less sodium.

Avoiding Food Addictions

An addiction is defined as a recurring compulsion by an individual to engage in some specific activity despite harmful consequences to the individual's health, mental state, or social life. Legal or illegal, an addiction can be a key risk factor for chronic disease and poor health. In a published paper on addictions Dr. James Forbes states, "Addictions don't wave off like flies. Once an addiction has gotten into one's flesh, mind, nervous system, brain, feet, and fingernails, from there it is a life-and-death struggle."

The battleground has become the mind and body. This territory has been possessed by the enemy of God and will not surrender without a fight. Addictions have a voice and a will. The person no longer speaks or hears the language of love. The innate wiring to God has been short-circuited.

Forbes continues, "It is not easy. The person pulls, then the addiction pulls back. An addiction can talk to a person like a natural man. It'll ask you, 'What do you mean, letting go? You can't get along without me! You do what I say you do.'" And so it is with food.

Sugar, fat, and meat are the most addictive of deceptive foods (Proverbs 23:1-3). We crave these foods and the body expects them. Some of these are habit-forming due to food additives like monosodium glutamate (MSG), which is a flavor and appetite enhancer. MSG is in food all over the world. Other deceptive ingredients include sodium, caffeine, alcohol, and nicotine.

To rid ourselves of the need for these foods, consider the following steps:

1. Ask the Father for help. Seek an understanding of what these foods do for you and why you eat them.

2. Consider a two or three day fresh vegetable juice fast using a juicer (kitchen appliance). If you do not have a juicer, you can purchase powder or tablets made of greens like barley, chlorella, spirulina, and wheat grass. These can be purchased at any health food or natural grocery store. Include a lot of room temperature water to help detoxify the body.

3. When you end your fast, start by eating homemade soups with fresh vegetables and grains, steamed vegetables, and salads.

4. Take a food supplement called spirulina in tablet form. Spirulina is a food supplement and can be taken without food. It has proven very effective in eliminating food cravings.

5. Read the labels on your food to make sure you are eating as purely as possible.

6. Exercise three days per week.

7. Continue to move forward with the other Disciplines of Wellness that we have discussed.

We must also avoid negative self-talk. For example, some of the popular support groups for addicts constantly have participants admit that they are addicts. This reminds every cell in the body to hold onto its need and demand for that addictive substance. It is putting a welcome mat out for the situation to always be there. It makes it easy to move from one addiction to another. God promises to help us when dealing with addictions and bad habits. There is nothing too hard for God to do. Resolve in your mind and within your heart that you want God to move this problem out of your life. And remember these Scriptures:

I Corinthians 6:19-20

Or didn't you realize that your body is a sacred place, the place of the Holy Spirit? Don't you see that you can't live however you please, squandering what God paid such a high price for? The physical part of you is not some piece of property belonging to the spiritual part of you. God owns the whole works. So let people see God in and through your body.

I Corinthians 10:13

No test or temptation that comes your way is beyond the course of what others have had to face. All you need to remember is that God will never let you down; he'll never let you be pushed past your limit; he'll always be there to help you come through it.

II Corinthians 10:4-5

We use our powerful God-tools for smashing warped philosophies, tearing down barriers erected against the truth of God, fitting every loose thought and emotion and impulse into the structure of life shaped by Christ.

Pure Is Sure

In a diseased culture, we are encouraged to eat foods that are tasty but empty of the healing nutrients needed by a strong, well body. Sugar (especially refined sugar) is being linked to obesity and other diseases. In the Book of Wisdom we are told, "When you're given a box of candy, don't gulp it all down; eat too much chocolate and you'll make yourself sick." There are many nonfood items being added to food. These items stabilize processed food. They help maintain color, taste, and shelf life. When we eat foods that are low in nutrients or foods that contain nonfood items, the body uses energy to process them even though they are of no benefit. These items have been used to extend the shelf life of foods, and as a result, retain profits. Terry Dorian suggests that we ask the following questions when food is before us:

1. **How close is the food to its original state?**
2. **What do the raw materials look like?**
3. **Why am I eating this food?**

Reading labels is important as we pursue wellness on God's terms. We must know what we are eating in order to make better choices.

Drinking Pure

The body is more than 80 percent water. In all of creation, God used water as a basic element. Water must be the first-choice beverage in order to maintain good health. The lack of water affects every part of our body, especially the brain. For a low-calorie drink, add lemon or a bit of fruit or vegetable juice. Avoid caffeinated beverages as they pull water out of the body. Suggested water intake:

Adults	Six to eight glasses per day (8 oz)
Children	Step 1: Divide your child's weight by 2 to get ounces
	Step 2: Divide ounces by 8 to get number of glasses

A large portion of added sugar in the American diet comes from the consumption of sugar-sweetened beverages. We are drinking our calories. The *Dietary Guidelines for Americans 2010* indicates that one way for people to reduce their intake of added sugars is to reduce the amount of sugar-sweetened beverages they drink. The consumption of sugar-sweetened beverages begins in early childhood and increases as children age. In 2002, the Feeding Infants and Toddlers Study (FITS) reported that 44 percent of toddlers ages 19–24 months old had consumed either fruit drinks (38 percent) or carbonated soda (11 percent) at least once a day.

A study using National Health and Nutrition Examination surveys found that overweight youths ages 2–19 years old consumed a higher proportion of their calories from carbonated soft drinks (regular and low calorie) and supplemental foods and beverages containing added sugar than their non-overweight counterparts.

In 2008, a Federal Trade Commission (FTC) study looked at the expenditures and activities of 44 companies that market food and beverages to children and adolescents. The study reported that in 2006, $474 million was directed at adolescents in the age range of 12 to 17. A significant portion, $116 million, was for school-based marketing. Much of the promotion focuses on children because of their increased spending power, purchasing influence, and future as adult consumers. These facts reinforce our need to limit the amount of access the media has to our children.

Let's face it: plain water has some stiff competition these days. Who wants water when you can get any beverage you can imagine, from colas to fruit juices to punches and drinks that are clear, sparkling, smooth, slushy, hot, cold, caffeinated, decaffeinated, with alcohol or without, regular or light? Better yet, who needs water? The answer: all of us! Drinking water is even more important when we consume these other drinks, most of which dehydrate us.

Did you know that the brain is 95 percent water, the lungs are 90 percent water, and blood is 83 percent water? Water is what nourishes and transports oxygen and nutrients to every organ and tissue in the body. Water also helps produce urine, which is how we eliminate all of the harmful substances that have been extracted from our blood. Although our kidneys will produce urine whether we drink water or not, lack of water requires our kidneys to work much harder.

We can live for about five weeks without protein, carbohydrates, and fats but only five days without water. Every day, the average adult body loses about three quarts of water. Some nutritionists estimate that as many as 80 percent of Americans are suffering from chronic dehydration.

Ideally, we should get most of our water as a result of eating high water-content foods such as fruits, vegetables, and their juices. However, most Americans eat mostly concentrated foods that have had the water removed from them by processing or cooking.

An average-size adult should drink at least eight glasses of pure water a day. A good way to determine how much water your body needs is to take your body weight and divide by two. Then drink that amount in ounces of water each day. For example, a five-foot, four-inch woman weighing approximately 130 pounds should consume 65 ounces, or eight 8-ounce glasses, of water each day.

Drinking water at room temperature is best. Cold drinks shock the system. Tap water is a good start. Let the tap run for a minute to clear stagnant water sitting in your pipes. If you have concerns about the safety of your water, have it tested by a lab.

Spring water is recommended over tap water because it is rich in minerals but low in additives like chlorine and fluoride. Distilled water is the purest form of water and is best for internal cleansing and during sickness.

Even a slight reduction of water in the body can affect our ability to think clearly, breathe properly, and have energy to function. If our body is made of mostly water and we never drink water to flush or replenish it, what we end up with is a swamp-like environment in the body. No one wants to live near a swamp and no one likes the thought of creating a swamp within his or her own body (dirt, odor, and toxins included).

According to Dr. Fereydoon Batmanghelidj, author of *Your Body's Many Cries for Water*, "Chronic pains in the body are often indicators of chronic dehydration." It has also been proven that many diseases start in the colon. Dr. Donnica Moore, a specialist in women's health, states: "Most people do not know that drinking eight glasses of water daily decreases the risk of colon cancer by 45 percent." Water helps transport solid wastes and toxins out of the body and aids in the elimination of these wastes through the colon. A diet that consists of fiber, high water-content foods, and water maintains a healthy colon. This type of diet along with water helps scrape the colon and prevents the clogging that causes disease.

The money it costs us every year for doctor visits and prescription drugs is phenomenal. Many of us, at one time, have admitted that we do not like drinking water. Think of water as a prescription that is administered by God. Add a slice of lemon. See drinking water as an investment in your body. It is the least expensive and most valuable prescription you will ever buy!

Healthy Eating Requires Thought and Planning

We discussed earlier that humans are born to instinctively know hunger. No one has to teach hunger. When we are hungry, we get grumpy, headachy, shaky, and lose the ability to think clearly. We know that hunger is coming, therefore common sense should teach us to anticipate the need for food and make provisions.

Before you go to the grocery store or farmer's market, decide what you would like to have available for breakfast each day and make a list of what you will need to purchase. Next, determine what you and your family will have for lunch each day. Add all the ingredients for lunch to your list. What will you have for dinner each night? Dinner can be used as leftovers for lunch or breakfast. Write that down. Next, think of the snacks you will need for each family member. Add that to your list. Once your list is complete, check your pantry to see what you already have on the list and adjust. Buy extra fruit and vegetables in season and freeze a portion of them for the winter. Appendix E has a sample weekly food planner to assist with this exercise.

Honoring God Motivates Us to Eat Well

Like moving, eating is an act of worship. The value that God puts on us should encourage us to see our bodies as the temples of the Holy Spirit He expects them to be (1 Corinthians 6:19). As we practice obedience to God's Word, we will see that it is our job to use the foods and the lifestyle outlined in Scripture to keep the body strong. We should want to provide ourselves the best food available and to eat in the most peaceful place. We want to avoid eating under stressful conditions, and we do not want to risk being under the influence of gluttonous eating or drinking. Sweets and too much meat cause disease and weaken the body.

There was a time that I absolutely hated to cook! Sugar—and a lot of it—was my comfort and seemed adequate enough for me to get by. A yogurt and cheese puffs for dinner after a long day at work was normal. If it came in a box with a few instructions like "Add ½ cup of water," that was my meal of choice. My body took this abuse for a long time. Eventually my body was not able to suppress the effect of my food choices and began to present ailments.

So how have I become such a wonderful cook? Love! It is not my love for cooking. It is realizing the high value God has for me. If I see my value then I need to care enough to nourish myself with the best food possible. I love my family enough to have their food minister to them holistically. That love is then transferred into every item I prepare. I'm praying and thinking good thoughts over it as I select, prepare, and serve the meal. Jesus spent a lot of time eating with people in their homes. Healthy food ministers to our bodies and emotional well-being. Feeling healthy supports healthy emotions. Food collection is not garbage collection. It is an act of appreciation and self-preservation that is a requirement for enjoying life. As I value the opportunity to live, I have no desire to be sick and distracted by preventable malfunctions of the body. So I want to know every ingredient that is in my food. I need to use food as medicine and the first line of defense to keep all systems working properly.

> You know the old saying, "First you eat to live, and then you live to eat"? Well, it may be true that the body is only a temporary thing, but that's no excuse for stuffing your body with food, or indulging it with sex. Since the Master honors you with a body, honor him with your body!
> —I Corinthians 6:13

Prayers of Change
Prayer to Move to the Original Diet

Father, I know now that the original diet is the diet that is best for me. I confess that I have gone along with the world's way of eating. I have put too much priority on food and have embraced the so-called foods that weaken my body. Forgive me of my food sins. Help me each day to move towards the fruits, vegetables, grains, herbs, beans, nuts, and seeds that you have so lovingly and scientifically created to keep me well, in Jesus' name. Amen.

Prayers to Eat for Wellness

Weight Loss

Dear God, I surrender my body and my weight loss to your divine care and love. Please forgive me for destructive eating and drinking habits. I ask you to remove all excess and unnecessary weight from my body. Return my body to its most healthy and balanced state. Help me not to succumb to the quick weight loss schemes, but to move forward with patience in knowledge, faith, and the truth about proper eating. Give me eating habits that support my health and life energy. Teach me to love my body according to your will and how to care for it from this day forth in Jesus' name. Amen.

Palate Change

Lord, please change my taste buds to like and desire those foods that help make me well in Jesus' name. Amen.

Access to Healthy Food

Lord, we pray for the food supply. Help us to seek pure foods and increase the supply and demand for them based on our obedience to you and our purchasing decisions in Jesus' name. Amen.

 Food is power.

 God's original diet gives us our first line of defense against disease.

THE
SOLDIER'S
ADVANCE

E arlier we discussed that life and death are two bookends. For children of God, death is seen as a promotion. It is often called a "home going," which is descriptive of our souls returning to the Father. Children of God believe that the body is the shell, which decays upon death, but life in the Spirit continues in the Lord. Jesus said, "I go to prepare a place for you . . . that where I am there ye may be also" (John 14:2-3, KJV). Like all of the other promises Jesus gave, this is a big one. Common sense should have us realize that if we are His children then of course He wants to lead us, protect us, and insure our ordained promotion.

Why are we discussing death in a book about wellness? I have observed that many Christians are paralyzed by the fear of death and as a result do not live well. The fear of death can inhibit us and cause us to avoid risks or not pursue our purpose.

At one point in my life, the fear of death was very strong and I avoided risks to the point where I could not fully embrace the work I felt I was created to do. The world sees death as something negative and encourages life extension by any means necessary.

Clearly I had a faith issue and was not using the truth with common sense. The more I spent time with God in obedience and embraced His promises and assurance for living, I realized that I feared disappointing Him more than I feared death. We know that Christ took care of death. Now we live for him.

I choose to live well and have put in place the disciplines that line up with the will of God who outlines how we remain in good health (Proverbs

14:27). I personally have no desire to live a long time and be miserable or heavily medicated. Living long is not the same as living well. Obedience to God's way ensures health, according to III John 1:2. "I wish above all things that thou mayest prosper and be in health, even as thy soul prospereth," meaning as I grow in obedience, my health should parallel the mind of Christ within me. And the Book of Wisdom assures me that "the way of the Lord is strength to the upright" (Proverbs 10:29, KJV). Bodies age but they do not have to be diseased. I realize that you may be reading this book with a diseased body or sickness. I speak peace to you. The Lord did not say "get yourself together and then come to me." All are loved and welcome. Jesus' love meets us right where we are. Obedience at the point of awareness is what is important. His grace and provision helps us in whatever state we find ourselves.

In II Corinthians 5:1-5, the Apostle Paul reminds us that bodies die. They do not, however, have to be sick, broken, or diseased. They can just stop! They can just shut down like a machine. When our assignment is complete in this world, we leave the body and get promoted to our permanent home with the Lord. And the legacy we leave will be of a soldier who was fit to follow God. The eulogy of a soldier in Christ's army is our life. When soldiers in Christ's army have completed their assignment, they will be promoted at the appointed time. We must remember the promise of God that if we believe in Jesus we will not perish but have everlasting life (John 3:16, KJV). The Apostle Paul reminds us that to be absent from the body is to be present with the Lord (II Corinthians 5:8, KJV).

The world sees death and associates it with loss. But we who are in the Kingdom see it as closing up shop in the physical so we can meet Jesus and live with him forever! For us, death is a quick, middle passage that leads to a deeper life with the Father in heaven, thanks to Jesus.

No one knows the exact time of promotion, however, good soldiers should have a sense of when most of their assignments are completed. The Apostle Paul knew, and Jesus knew.

Whether God promotes through physical death or comes back to relieve us, everyone in the Kingdom will be relocated to heaven to be with the trinity of God! This is the hope and excitement we have—knowing that life does not end in this world. The best and great celebration is yet to come! Here are the words of the Apostle and Pastor Paul from I Thessalonians 4:13-14 (NLT):

> "And now, dear brothers and sisters, we want you to know what will happen to the believers who have died so you will not grieve like people who have no hope. For since we believe that Jesus died and was raised to life again, we also believe that when Jesus returns, God will bring back with Him the believers who have died."

Many in the Kingdom refer to physical death as a departure. I see it as a promotion and time of rest until that great day. The funeral service for a soldier should be more celebratory than sad!

We must ask the Father to help us walk the path of life without the presence of our dear loved one. Although the assignment of our dearly departed one is done, our assignment on earth is not. So provision will be made for us to move ahead and stay well as we seek clarity for life without that loved one.

Many soldiers do not have the spiritual maturity to anticipate their departures and meet Jesus in their new home. The world and those who love it are already spiritually dead and view this physical existence as something to hold on to for as long as possible. We want to be present with the Lord. Bodies may die but people do not. The Apostle Paul encourages us to press on in the Book of Philippians, "I focus on this one thing: forgetting the past and looking forward to what lies ahead, I press on to reach the end of the race and receive the heavenly prize for which God, through Christ Jesus, is calling us" (3:13-14, NLT).

Parting Decisions

In my book *Got Cancer? Congratulations! Now You Can Start Living* I outline the stewardship needed to prepare for being promoted. One of our final acts of love for your family is to ensure that you have stated your wishes and made provisions for handling your remains, including your body and estate.

There are two tasks that I recommend for a soldier of God: write a living will and a last will and testament. These two documents eliminate the confusion around your promotion.

The **living will** simply states whether or not you want to be resuscitated and put on life support machines. This choice is yours to make. In the absence of a living will, the family has the burden of choosing. Personally speaking, if I cannot breathe on my own, I believe it is because the Father has allowed breath to leave my body. It is not up to anyone to attempt to bring it back! We must make our own decisions.

The **last will and testament** is a document that many feel is for the rich and famous. But if you do not complete one, depending on where you live, your death can become a hardship and very painful for your survivors. Here are some topics to include in your last will and testament:

- ❖ Assign someone to carry out your will.
- ❖ State funeral/burial preferences.
- ❖ Assign possessions (houses, cars, money, insurance policies, and pensions).
- ❖ Set up scholarships, trusts, causes, and organizations.

Our society has made it necessary to explicitly state what happens to your estate after you are promoted. Scripture does admonish us to leave an inheritance to our grandchildren (Proverbs 13:22). From a stewardship perspective, it would be good to transfer your earthly goods to others in your life.

For examples of a living will and last will and testament, visit LawDepot.com or other law website.

 If God has scheduled my expiration, I should see each day as a good thing.

 As a child of God, I do not fear death. Death is a promotion.

CONCLUSION: THE CATALYST FOR WELLNESS

L iving well is not about being skinny, handsome, gorgeous, rich, or the picture of health. It's not about fitting into that size eight dress to attend a high school reunion. Living long is not the same as living well.

Embracing God, seeing your value, and knowing your purpose (which is the work God has planned to do through you) should be the motivating factors to care for yourself. Falling in love with God through Christ is the stimulus to change. We want to be the best we can be. We want to make Him proud. As you grow in your primary care relationship with God the Creator and Father, you will see that taking care of yourself by practicing the essential principles of wellness is a must in order for you to accomplish your great work. Taking care of yourself is also demonstrating the love you have for God and an expression of your appreciation for Him making you. You are a one-of-a-kind designer original, never again to grace this world. Living well is your lifestyle.

As I have said before, life and death are two bookends in time. The chapters within those bookends are wonderfully developed as we see that we are a part of a large tapestry that is needed in order to meet the needs for the greater good (glorifying God). Our story is written based on how we reflect the intended plan of God for our physical existence.

This is the motivation that allows us to close this book and begin the move toward wellness. You may or may not find a lot of positive reinforcement for many of these disciplines. There are many reasons for this, the most prevalent reason being that misery and disobedience love company. **The fellowship of the miserable can railroad any attempt you make at**

taking better care of yourself and your loved ones. You will also find the fire hose of stress waiting for the opportunity to push your back to the wall and revert you to your old familiar habits. They may not be good but they are comfortable. Know that, moment by moment, you have the opportunity to make a decision that is much different from the decision you made moments before it. Confessing your shortcomings to the Father empowers you to forgive yourself and try again. You have the ability to affirm yourself and press forward to a new beginning.

Your assignment from God is unique, fulfilling, and specially prepared for you. Your intended purpose is the key factor that helps you recognize your value and provides the motivation and determination you've been lacking to live well. No longer does your body have a need to self-destruct. It is a beautiful one-of-a-kind temple, totally illuminated, and energized by the very God of all that is! You've got wonderful work to do!

Wellness is about what you receive from God so that you can give. If you love someone, you want to spend time with him or her. God loves us and desires more than anything to spend time with us. It is difficult to keep promises to people if they won't spend time with you. It is hard to give the gifts of joy, peace, protection, and encouragement if they do not acknowledge your existence in their lives. It is also a challenge to support someone who has no confidence or expectation that you are able to do it.

We have become aware of the impact being in a diseased culture has on our ability to be healthy. We can put our intelligence back in God's hands to bring forth the plan for restoring our health and making it a plan that is doable and individualized for each of us. I pray blessings upon your life as you move to your distinctively designed path with wellness as your lifestyle.

A wellness lifestyle does not mean you will never be sick. The consequences of our choices can take their course. God is a God of correction and forgiveness. According to Scripture, He does not keep us from all afflictions, but uses them to demonstrate His faithfulness and love, just as parents correct their dear children (Job 5:19). Arthur Pink, author of *The Attributes of God,* states, "To be full of care, to view our situation with dark forebodings, to anticipate the morrow with sad anxiety, is to reflect poorly upon the faithfulness of God. He who has heard our prayers in the past will not refuse to supply your needs in the present emergency." God's Word in Job 5:17-19 speaks to this also: "So, what a blessing when God steps in and corrects you! Mind you, don't despise the discipline of Almighty God! True, He wounds, but He also dresses the wound; the same hand that hurts you, heals you. From one disaster after another He delivers you; no matter what the calamity, the evil can't touch you."

Finally, I pray that our God, who fed the warrior Elijah (I Kings 19:5-8) from heaven, will send whatever your trinity is in need of (whether it be healing, longevity, or wellness) to complete your life's purpose. Keep your coordinates rooted in the Word of God and listen for His instructions. With your wellness disciplines, He will protect the investment He has made in you. May everything good from God our Father be yours (Colossians 1:1). Live deeply. Live well!

And let me live whole and holy, soul and body, so I can always walk with my head held high. —Psalm 119:80

Recap of the Seven Disciplines of Wellness

1. Pursue Primary Care
- ❖ Essential for wellness.
- ❖ Because God cares for me and I care for Him, I can care for others and myself.
- ❖ Primary care is God's love moving in and through me as I pursue Him.

2. Maintain Good Communication
- ❖ A prayer life is essential to God's plan for wellness.
- ❖ The prayer framework helps build a life of prayer.
- ❖ Only way to know the *you* that you were created to be and have the power to be it!

3. Be Intentional About Life
- ❖ Avoid distractions and addictions.
- ❖ Remember our value to God.
- ❖ Know the provision for fulfillment and completion.

4. Use Common Sense
- ❖ Study Scripture to know the truth and how to think.
- ❖ Embrace the mind of Christ within.
- ❖ Use God's weapons to correct and protect your thought life.

5. Establish a Sacred Place to Live
- ❖ Home should be more peaceful than any place outside.
- ❖ Home is my healing station, the place where I nurture wellness.
- ❖ Home is the root structure for Kingdom culture.

6. Move
- ❖ The body was made "to do" and "to be."
- ❖ A fit body reflects the indwelling of the Holy Spirit of God, the "doer" of His will.

7. Eat and Drink Real Food
- ❖ Based on biblical principles; pursue real food, which is the original diet.
- ❖ Use food as medicine.
- ❖ God's plan to sustain the body.

Appendix A: Prayers for a Wellness Lifestyle

Restoration

Father, we thank you for life. Thank you that every breath we take is the receipt of a perfect gift from you. We breathe in the hope, excitement, and energy that it brings. We exhale the waste from our body, mind, and spirit. We release the need to carry waste in our bodies. We use our imagination to see every cell in our bodies receiving the oxygen and food that restores our DNA to its corrected state. Every cell in my body yields to your will, your way for your glory. I remember that the joy of the Lord is my strength. Thank you that my heart pumps joy and my lungs receive life and hope in Jesus' name. Amen.

Fear

I have the ultimate protection in the full armor of God, so I have no fear of being harmed as I move about. You have not given me the spirit of fear, but of power, and of love, and of a sound mind. I also have the fruit of the spirit, which proves your presence in my life. That presence changes the atmosphere wherever I go, so even my enemies are at peace with me. I can expect you to prepare a table for me in the midst of my enemies. Amen.

Forgiveness

Father, please reveal all sin in my life that is separating me from you. I want to agree with you. I hate sin also. Forgive me, Lord, in the name of Jesus. Amen.

Changing Eating Habits

Father, please correct my palate and taste buds to desire the foods I need to eat in order to be healthy in Jesus' name. Amen.

Purpose

Father, in Jesus' name, we thank you for letting us know that you have a plan for each of us. We are all designer originals and you watched us form from nothing in the womb to a whole person with purpose.

I pray that you would help me understand my unique work, for it is that work that justifies my existence. You have made provision for everything I need to live intentionally, complete my assignment, and bring glory to your name.

I have the ultimate protection in the full armor of God, so I have no fear of being harmed as I move about, being focused and doing my work. I am fully supported and your joy strengthens me. I like where you are taking me. It is well. Even though it is not my will, please let your purpose be completed through me. Thank you, in Jesus' name. Amen.

Smoker's Prayer

Father, you are all-powerful and wonderful in all of your ways. I confess my sins and ask for forgiveness in Jesus' name. I lay before you my habit of smoking which is a disgrace against the body that you have asked me to care for. I know that habits impact my mind and spirit as well. My entire trinity has the expectation of a smoke and my body has become dependent. I have attempted to stop, but I confess that I have the desire and fairly enjoy smoking.

I know now that smoking impacts my ability to breathe and you are the controller of my breath. So in the name of Jesus, your dear son, please remove the desire, expectation, dependency, craving, and taste. I cannot do this without your help. Help me to see and run through the open doors that you will place on my path to help me escape. This is a miracle and I receive this deliverance. I will not try to do this myself as in the past. Help me to flow with your way. Amen.

> Because you have satisfied me, God, I promise to do everything you say.
> —Psalm 119:57

Appendix B: Time Log

Regaining control of our time starts with understanding that time is a gift and must be allocated properly. Complete the following time log for a typical weekday and a weekend day. After you have completed the time log, what truths have you discovered about the use of your time? How much time is allocated to relaxing with the television or surfing the Web? Can you use that time more wisely? Remember to include times that you exercised and notes on what healthy and unhealthy foods you ate.

Date (weekday): _____

Activities	Time Started	Time Spent
Woke Up		
Breakfast		
Lunch		
Dinner		
Sleep		
Total Hours		24 hours

Date (weekend): _____

Activities	Time Started	Time Spent
Woke Up		
Breakfast		
Lunch		
Dinner		
Sleep		
Total Hours		24 hours

Appendix C: Natural Household Cleaners

Aguirre, Sarah. "3 Homemade Natural Cleaning Products." About.com Housekeeping. Accessed January 19, 2012. http://housekeeping.about.com/cs/environment/a/alternateclean.htm.

Steinman David, and R. Michael Wisner. Living Healthy in a Toxic World, New York: The Berkley Publishing Group, 1996.

Zima Health Research Labs, www.zimahealth.com, 2011.

Appendix D: Sources of Calcium

Food, Standard Amount	Calcium (mg)	Calories
Fortified ready-to-eat cereals (various), 1 oz	236-1043	88-106
Soy beverage, calcium fortified, 1 cup	368	98
Sardines, Atlantic, in oil, drained, 3 oz	325	177
Tofu, firm, ½ cup	253	88
Pink salmon, canned, with bone, 3 oz	181	118
Collards, cooked from frozen, ½ cup	178	31
Molasses, blackstrap, 1 Tbsp	172	47
Spinach, cooked from frozen, ½ cup	146	30
Soybeans, green, cooked, ½ cup	130	127
Turnip greens, cooked from frozen, ½ cup	124	24
Ocean perch, Atlantic, cooked, 3 oz	116	103
Oatmeal, plain and flavored, instant, fortified, 1 packet prepared	99-110	97-157
Cowpeas, cooked, ½ cup	106	80
White beans, canned, ½ cup	96	153
Kale, cooked from frozen, ½ cup	90	20
Okra, cooked from frozen, ½ cup	88	26
Soybeans, mature, cooked, ½ cup	88	149
Blue crab, canned, 3 oz	86	84
Beet greens, cooked from fresh, ½ cup	82	19
Pak-choi, Chinese cabbage, cooked from fresh, ½ cup	79	10
Clams, canned, 3 oz	78	126
Dandelion greens, cooked from fresh, ½ cup	74	17
Rainbow trout, farmed, cooked, 3 oz	73	144

Source: Nutrient values from Agricultural Research Service (ARS) Nutrient Database for Standard Reference, Release 17. Foods are from ARS single nutrient reports, sorted in descending order by nutrient content in terms of common household measures. Food items and weights in the single nutrient reports are adapted from those in 2002 revision of USDA Home and Garden Bulletin No. 72, Nutritive Value of Foods. Mixed dishes and multiple preparations of the same food item have been omitted from this table.

Recommended Dietary Allowances (RDAs) for Calcium

Age	Male	Female	Pregnant	Lactating
0-6 months*	200 mg	200 mg		
7-12 months*	260 mg	260 mg		
1-3 years	700 mg	700 mg		
4-8 years	1,000 mg	1,000 mg		
9-13 years	1,300 mg	1,300 mg		
14-18 years	1,300 mg	1,300 mg	1,300 mg	1,300 mg
19-50 years	1,000 mg	1,000 mg	1,000 mg	1,000 mg
51-70 years	1,000 mg	1,200 mg		
71+ years	1,200 mg	1,200 mg		

* Adequate Intake (AI)
Source: Office of Dietary Supplements, National Institutes of Health, Aug 2011

Appendix E: Weekly Food Planner

	Breakfast	Lunch	Dinner	Snacks
Mon				
Tue				
Wed				
Thu				
Fri				
Sat				
Sun				

Notes:

_____

_____

_____

Bibliography

Our Struggle for Wellness: The War

Centers for Disease Control and Prevention. *National Vital Statistics Reports: Deaths: Preliminary Data for 2009.* http://www.cdc.gov/nchs/data/nvsr/nvsr59/nvsr59_04.pdf.

Pilzer, Paul Z. *The New Wellness Revolution.* Hoboken, NJ: John Wiley & Sons, Inc., 2007.

Wellness Is a Lifestyle

Mayer, Diane P. *The Everything Health Guide to Controlling Anxiety.* Avon, MA: F+W Publications, 2005.

Ponder, Catherine. *The Dynamic Laws of Healing.* Camarillo, CA: DeVorss & Company, 1972.

The Wellness Battle Plan

Allen, Charles L. *God's Psychiatry.* Grand Rapids: Revell, 1997.

Bailey, Regina. "10 Facts About Cells." About.com Biology. Accessed January 19, 2012. http://biology.about.com/od/cellbiology/a/cells-facts.htm.

Balch, Phyllis A. *Prescription for Nutritional Healing.* 4th ed. New York: Avery, 2006.

Mayo Clinic. "High blood pressure (hypertension)." Last modified March 22, 2011. http://www.mayoclinic.com/health/high-blood-pressure/DS00100/DSECTION=risk-factors.

McWilliams, Peter. *You Can't Afford the Luxury of a Negative Thought.* Revised ed. N.p.: Mary Book, 1995.

National Institute of Mental Health. "Statistics." Last modified September 5, 2008. http://wwwapps.nimh.nih.gov/health/statistics/index.shtml.

Nightingale, Earl. *The Strangest Secret.* Read by the author. N.p.: Keys Company, 1999. Compact disc.

PBS Online. "Deadly Diseases: Malnutrition." Last modified March 2006.
http://www.pbs.org/wgbh/rxforsurvival/series/diseases/malnutrition.html.

Ponder, Catherine. *The Dynamic Laws of Healing*. Camarillo, CA: DeVorss &
Company, 1972.

Tolson, Chester L., and Harold G. Koenig. *The Healing Power of Prayer*. Grand
Rapids: Baker Books, 2004.

WebMD. "Causes of High Blood Pressure." Last modified March 6, 2009.
http://www.webmd.com/hypertension-high-blood-pressure/guide/blood-pressure-
causes.

Wood, Larry. Bible doctrine news. Accessed January 19, 2012.
http://www.biblenews1.com/beliefs.htm.

World Health Organization. "Mental health." Accessed January 24, 2012.
http://www.who.int/topics/mental_health/en.

Discipline 1: Pursue Primary Care
Lea, Larry. *Could You Not Tarry One Hour?*, Florida: Creation House, 1987.

Discipline 2: Maintain Good Communication
Baron, Kelly G., Kathryn J. Reid, Andrew S. Kern, and Phyllis C. Zee. "Behavior
and Psychology: Role of Sleep Timing in Caloric Intake and BMI." *Obesity* 19 (July
2011):1374-1381. doi:10.1038/oby.2011.100.

Bach, James F., Stengler, Mark, *Prescription for Natural Cures*, New Jersey: Wiley &
Sons, 2004.

Emsellem, Helene A. *Snooze... or Lose!* Washington, DC: Joseph Henry Press, 2006.

Got Questions Ministries. "What is the meaning of Christian worship?" Accessed
January 19, 2012. http://www.gotquestions.org/Christian-worship.html.

Goulart, Frances S. *Super Immunity Foods*. New York: McGraw-Hill, 2009.

National Sleep Foundation. "Sleep Hygiene." Accessed January 19, 2012. http://www.sleepfoundation.org/article/ask-the-expert/sleep-hygiene.

Summers, Kathy. "Keep Your Family Healthy." *Natural Health Magazine*. Accessed January 19, 2012. http://www.naturalhealthmag.com/health/keep-your-family-healthy.

Tolson, Chester L., and Harold G. Koenig. *The Healing Power of Prayer*. Grand Rapids: Baker Books, 2004.

Discipline 3: Be Intentional About Life
Frankl, Victor. *Man's Search for Meaning*. Boston: Beacon Press, 2006.

Rebecca Ray, Milla Sanes, John Schmitt. Center for Economic and Policy Research. "No Vacation Nation Revisited." Last modified May 2013. http://www.cepr.net/index.php/publications/reports/no-vacation-nation-2013.

Rebecca Ray, Janet C. Gornick, John Schmitt. Center for Economic and Policy Research. "Parent Leave Policies in 21 Countries: Assessing Generosity and Gender Equality." Last modified September 2008. http://www.cepr.net/index.php/publications/reports/plp/.

Discipline 4: Establish a Sacred Place to Live
Centers for Disease Control and Prevention. "Insufficient Sleep Is a Public Health Epidemic." Last modified March 17, 2011. http://www.cdc.gov/features/dsSleep.

Creative Home Decorating Room by Room. Accessed January 19, 2012. http://www.home-decorating-room-by-room.com.

Genovese, Stacy. "New Fume-Free Paint." *Good Housekeeping*. Last modified May 13, 2010. http://www.goodhousekeeping.com/product-reviews/research-institute/no-or-low-voc-paints.

Institute of Medicine. *Sleep Disorders and Sleep Deprivation: An Unmet Public Health Problem*. Washington, D.C.: The National Academies Press, 2006.

Science Daily. "The Top Five Actions Parents Can Take to Reduce Child Exposure to Toxic Chemicals at Home." Last modified June 15, 2011. http://www.sciencedaily.com/releases/2011/06/110615171402.htm.

Mary Madden, Amanda Lenhart, Maeve Duggan, Sandra Cortesi, Urs Gasser, The Pew Research Center, *Teens and Technology 2013*, March 13, 2013. http://www.pewinternet.org/Reports/2013/Teens-and-Tech/Summary-of-Findings/Overview.aspx.

Discipline 5: Use Common Sense
Haas, Elson. *Staying Healthy with the Seasons*. Berkeley, CA: Celestial Arts, 2003.

Lea, Larry. *Releasing the Prayer Anointing*. Nashville: Thomas Nelson, 1996.

Balch, Phyllis A. *Prescription for Nutritional Healing*. 4TH ED. New York: Avery, 2006./

Discipline 6: Move
Centers for Disease Control and Prevention. "Chronic Disease and Health Promotion." Last modified July 7, 2010. http://www.cdc.gov/chronicdisease/overview/index.htm.

Centers for Disease Control and Prevention. Database of State Legislative and Regulatory Action to Prevent Obesity and Improve Nutrition and Physical Activity. Accessed July 1, 2009. http://apps.nccd.cdc.gov/DNPALeg.

Winslow, Ron. "Watching TV Linked to Higher Risk of Death." *Wall Street Journal*. Last modified January 12, 2010. http://online.wsj.com/article/SB10001424052748704055104574652340708172608.html.

Discipline 7: Eat and Drink Real Food
American Heart Association. "Fish and Omega-3 Fatty Acids." Last modified September 7, 2010. http://www.heart.org/HEARTORG/GettingHealthy/NutritionCenter/HealthyDietGoals/Fish-and-Omega-3-Fatty-Acids_UCM_303248_Article.jsp#.Txhb6vmo9I0.

American Heart Association. "Frequently Asked Questions About Sugar." Last modified May 25, 2010. http://www.heart.org/HEARTORG/GettingHealthy/NutritionCenter/HealthyDietGoals/Frequently-Asked-Questions-About-Sugar_UCM_306725_Article.jsp#.TxhdZPmo9I0.

Balch, Phyllis A. *Prescription for Nutritional Healing*. 4th ed. New York: Avery, 2006.
Batmanghelidj, Fereydoon. *Your Body's Many Cries for Water*. Vienna, VA: Global Health Solutions, 2008.

Centers for Disease Control and Prevention. "Behavioral Risk Factor Surveillance System Prevalence Trends and Data: Nationwide (States, DC, and Territories) - 2007." Accessed January 19, 2012. http://apps.nccd.cdc.gov/brfss/page.asp?yr=2007&state=US&cat=FV#FV.

Centers for Disease Control and Prevention. "Protein." Last modified October 31, 2011. http://www.cdc.gov/nutrition/everyone/basics/protein.html.

The China Study. "About The China Study." Accessed January 19, 2012. http://thechinastudy.com.

DeHaan, M.R. *The Chemistry of the Blood*. Grand Rapids: Zondervan, 1983.

Division of Nutrition and Physical Activity. Research to Practices Series No. 3: Does Drinking Beverages with Added Sugars Increase the Risk of Overweight? Atlanta: Centers for Disease Control and Prevention, 2006.

Dorian, Terry. *Health Begins in Him*. Lafayette, LA: Vital Issues Press, 1995.

The Environmental Working Group. "EWG's 2-11 Shopper's Guide to Pesticides in Produce." Accessed January 19, 2012. http://www.ewg.org/foodnews.

Foodconsumer.org. "EAFUS: A Food Additive Database." Last modified on April 23, 2008. Accessed April 20, 2011. http://foodconsumer.org/7777/8888/F_ood_C_hemicals_37/042302422008_EAFUS_A_Food_Additive_Database.shtml.

Foodpolitics.com. *Breaking Down The Chain: A Guide to the Soft Drink Industry*, National Policy & Legal Analysis Network to Prevent Childhood Obesity, 2011.

Forbes, James. "A Word About Addictions." *Biblical Strategies for a Community in Crisis*, edited by Colleen Birchett. Chicago: Urban Ministries, 1992.

Jordan, Surina Ann. "Plate for a Plant-Based Diet." Annapolis, MD: Zima Health Research Labs, 2011.

Mayo Clinic. "Dietary fats: Know which types to choose." Last modified February 15, 2011. http://www.mayoclinic.com/health/fat/NU00262.

Meat Science at Texas A&M University. "Kosher and Halal." Accessed January 19, 2012. http://meat.tamu.edu/kosher.html.

Moore, Donnica. "The Health Benefits of Drinking Water." DrDonnica.com. Last modified October 21, 2003. http://www.drdonnica.com/today/00007230.htm. Nutritional Epidemiology Branch, Division of Cancer Epidemiology and Genetics, National Cancer Institute, National Institutes of Health, Department of Health and Human Services, Bethesda, MD, U.S.A.

Organic.org. "The 'Dirty Dozen.'" Accessed January 19, 2012. http://www.organic.org/articles/showarticle/article-214.

Pitchford, Paul. *Healing With Whole Foods*. 3rd ed. Berkeley, CA: North Atlantic Books, 2002.

U.S. Department of Health and Human Services and U.S. Department of Agriculture. *Dietary Guidelines for Americans, 2010*. 7th ed. Washington, DC: U.S. Government Printing Office, January 2011.

U.S. Department of Veterans Affairs. MOVE! page. Last modified July 27, 2011. http://www.move.va.gov.

U.S. National Library of Medicine. "Foods - fresh vs. frozen or canned." MedlinePlus. Last modified October 22, 2011. http://www.nlm.nih.gov/medlineplus/ency/article/002095.htm.

Van Straten, Michael. *The Healthy Food Directory*. Barnes & Noble Books, 1999.

Yamamoto, Shigeru, et al. "Can dietary supplementation of monosodium glutamate improve the health of the elderly?" *The American Journal of Clinical Nutrition* 90, no. 3 (Sept. 2009): 844S-849S. http://www.ajcn.org/content/90/3/844S.full.

Zeratsky, Katherine. "Are high-protein diets safe for weight loss?" Mayo Clinic. Last modified June 19, 2010. http://www.mayoclinic.com/health/high-protein-diets/AN00847.

The Soldier's Advance
LawDepot.com. "Last Will and Testament" and "Living Will." Accessed October 2, 2013. http://www.lawdepot.com/contracts/groups/estate.

Conclusion: The Catalyst for Wellness
Jordan, Surina Ann. *Got Cancer? Congratulations! Now You Can Start Living*. Bloomington, IN: Author House, 2003.

Pink, Arthur W. *The Attributes of God*, Radford, VA: Wilder Publications, 2009.

Index

abuse – 27, 40, 44, 78, 112, 140
accept Christ – 19, 20, 21, 51, 60
accountability – 32, 52, 55, 105
act of worship – 59, 139
Adam and Eve – 18, 56
addiction – 83, 133-135, 149
addicts – 134
adolescents – 137
argumentativeness -- 45
alcohol – 39, 89, 130, 134, 137
all-knowing – 16, 68
all-powerful – 16, 28, 68, 151
allergic reaction – 99
ambassadors – 66
American diet – 119, 123, 136
American Heart Association – 109, 130, 132
ammunition – 92, 104
angelic ecstasy – 62
anger – 28, 34, 45, 51, 74, 96, 100, 101
animalistic – 36, 47
anti-wellness – 35
anxiety – 34, 45, 111, 147
Apostle Paul – 54, 62, 70, 86, 113, 121, 143, 144
appreciation – 96, 140, 146
approach – 6, 19, 46, 53, 92
armor of God – 25, 26, 27, 70, 150, 151
Arthur Pink -- 147
artificial sweeteners – 119
assignment – 64, 74, 83, 84, 88, 112, 143, 144, 147, 151
atmosphere – 31, 71, 93, 95, 98, 150
attacks – 24, 27, 33
attributes of God – 29
The Attributes of God – 147
authentic – 20, 24, 27, 30, 34, 56, 57, 60, 66, 82
aversion – 24
avoidance – 89
awareness – 25, 51, 61, 75, 90, 132, 143
baby – 15, 44, 58, 62
bad fat – 119, 124, 131
balance – 6, 87, 91, 100, 104, 110, 111, 141
battle – 10, 11, 18, 21-25, 28, 31-34, 43, 46, 49, 54, 70, 90, 92, 110, 112, 133
beans – 46, 118, 125, 126, 128, 130, 140, 155
big business – 13, 37
blood sugar – 44, 46, 78, 118, 128, 129
boredom – 47
brain – 24, 34, 35, 36, 37, 38, 46, 47, 51, 77, 99, 104, 119, 133, 136, 137
breakfast – 139, 152, 153, 156
brick and mortar – 60
bridge – 18, 21, 31
brown bag – 63
Burt Bacharach – 18
buying behaviors – 13
caffeine – 46, 78, 134
calcium – 121, 128, 130, 155
Caleb -- 110
calendar – 96
calm – 34, 64, 97, 100, 103
calories – 78, 114, 131, 132, 136, 137, 155
cancer – 10, 12, 97, 108, 117, 119, 121, 138, 144

capacity – 37, 38, 40, 42, 46, 71, 76, 105, 108, 110-112, 132
carbohydrate – 48, 125, 128, 132, 137
caregiver – 46, 58, 68
catastrophes – 37
Catherine Ponder – 16, 34
CDC – 12, 103, 132
cells – 43, 77, 118, 123
cellular level – 120
chaos – 38, 47
chemical – 24, 41, 51, 58, 97, 101, 115, 116, 119, 131
Chester Tolson – 43, 68, 74, 83
children of God – 9, 25, 29, 30, 31, 52, 79, 84, 99, 142
children of Israel – 56, 117, 118
China Study – 117, 121
chlorophyll – 117, 120, 128
choice – 6, 16-25, 33, 37, 38, 42, 52, 72, 89, 122, 145, 147
cholesterol – 110, 124, 129, 130
chronic dehydration – 137, 138
chronic disease – 12, 15, 16, 46, 47, 89, 108, 118, 121, 123, 129, 133
chronic stress – 41, 43-45, 48, 67
church – 60, 64, 65, 76, 90, 91, 94
clean air – 95, 97
clear thinking – 16, 32
clenched jaws – 45
coach – 25, 57
cocoon for healing – 95
cognitive – 37
color – 36, 50, 95, 99, 100, 102-104, 136
commandment – 55, 56, 57, 61, 84
commit – 29, 38, 47, 72, 79, 80, 92, 112
common area – 101, 104
common sense – 6, 7, 10, 14-17, 19, 27, 29, 32, 37, 52, 54, 64, 71, 89, 90, 92, 94, 102, 108, 117, 120, 122, 125, 126, 129, 139, 142, 149
communication – 6, 65, 68, 70, 95, 96, 99, 105, 149
communion – 17, 27, 65, 99, 125
community groups – 13
companies – 12, 14, 115, 137
compare – 36, 42, 59, 133
conduit for love – 65
conflict – 31, 64, 65, 84
confusion – 12, 21, 31, 41, 145
counter attack – 33, 34, 35, 37-39, 41, 45, 46, 48, 50, 51
counterfeit god – 17
creation – 11, 17, 18, 23, 30, 33, 104, 122, 136
creator – 16, 17, 21, 28, 30, 34, 36, 50, 58, 80, 146
critical of others – 45
crucifixion – 19
daily defense – 75
daily renewal – 73, 74, 112
Daniel – 120
death – 11, 12, 18, 19, 20, 22, 47, 49, 50, 51, 54, 65, 94, 119, 133, 142-145
deceptive food – 118, 120, 121, 126, 134
dependability – 64
depravity – 121
depression – 45, 83, 100, 108, 124

destroyer – 24, 63
destruction – 23, 24, 52, 90, 122
destructive behavior – 24, 37, 83
detoxify – 110, 118, 129, 134
Devil – 25, 75
devitalized – 119
diabetes – 12, 16, 78, 108, 117, 119, 120
Diane Peters Mayer – 18
dietary guidelines – 129, 132, 136
dietary plan – 121
digestive – 115, 118, 132
dinner – 48, 76, 78, 123, 139, 140, 152, 153, 156
Dionne Warwick – 18
discipline – 51-54
discouragement – 50, 86
diseased culture – 6, 11-14, 18, 20-22, 28, 30, 34, 38, 40, 42, 46, 50-53, 61, 64, 70, 71, 85, 87, 94, 95, 114, 121, 122, 135, 147
disobedience – 24, 33, 50, 55, 56, 146
DNA -122, 150
Donnica Moore – 138
drinking water – 53, 137-139
drugs – 46, 89, 138
dyes – 115, 119
Earl Nightingale – 37
earth – 16, 17, 20, 30, 31, 36, 50, 54, 69, 70, 79, 85, 91, 117, 118, 144, 145
eat to live – 46, 140
eating disorders – 45
Elijah – 126, 148
Elson Haas – 89
emotional injury – 40, 47
emotionally toxic – 64
enemy – 18, 21-27, 31-35, 38, 39, 46, 47, 50, 52, 59, 62, 65, 75, 82, 86, 90, 114, 119, 122, 125, 133
enlisted – 25, 92
environment – 7, 32, 58, 61, 63-65, 93, 95, 97-103, 106, 116, 123, 138
Environmental Working Group – 116
eulogy – 14
evidence-based story – 19
executor – 18, 43, 94
expectation – 15, 27, 28, 38, 59, 65, 68, 82, 104, 147, 151
faith – 7, 26-28, 30, 39, 41, 42, 48, 49, 62, 70, 72, 74, 76, 80, 84, 94, 96, 100, 141, 142, 147, 148
family history – 15
family meal – 63, 101
famine – 126
farm – 63, 114, 115, 120, 129, 139, 155
farmer's market – 139
fat – 45, 48, 77, 110, 112, 115, 119, 121, 128-132, 134
fear – 13, 34, 35, 37, 39, 42, 45, 47, 49, 50, 52, 57, 64, 74, 87, 99, 142, 145, 150, 151
Federal Trade Commission – 137
Feeding Infants and Toddlers study – 136
feeding people – 63
Fereydoon Batmanghelidj – 138
fiber – 82, 118, 121, 124, 128, 138
fiery darts – 26, 27
fight-or-flight – 44
fish – 46, 98, 109, 117, 119, 125, 126, 128, 130, 131
fitness industry – 109
flavorings – 119

Food and Drug Administration – 115
food as medicine – 140, 149
food fads – 120
food labels – 115, 134, 136
food photography – 37
food preparation – 63
food supplement – 134
food supply – 61, 115, 119, 122, 131, 132, 141
forgiveness – 20, 25, 42, 51, 70, 92, 112, 147, 150, 151
formulas – 69
foundation for wellness – 16
framework – 18, 30, 32, 52, 55, 70, 71, 76, 77, 80, 105, 149
freedom – 27, 52, 61, 92, 105, 122
fruit – 41, 48, 79, 99, 106, 114, 115, 117, 118, 120, 123, 125, 128, 129, 136, 137, 139, 140
fruit of the spirit – 150
garden – 63, 96, 117, 120, 155
genetic code – 32
genetically modified organism (GMO) – 115, 122
gentle spirit – 64
gentleness – 49
God is love – 16
God's Psychiatry – 33
God's reflection – 64
good fat – 45, 128, 131
goodness – 42, 49, 72, 92, 94
government – 13, 65, 90
grace – 32, 68, 69, 71, 73, 143, 146, 151
grapefruit seed extract – 116
grateful heart technique – 34
gratitude – 49, 59, 72, 94
greater good – 11, 40, 51, 60, 83, 84, 88, 146
grinding teeth -- 45
grocery store – 31, 134, 13
growing older – 39
growth hormone – 115
Harold Koenig – 43
headaches – 45
healer – 63, 73
healing agents – 129
healing chambers – 96, 102
healing station – 95, 107, 149
health industry – 13
healthiest people – 30, 121
healthy images – 42
healthy mind – 23, 32-34, 49
healthy relationships – 32, 42, 105
healthy spirit – 23, 40, 49, 50
healthy thoughts – 90
health care – 13
helmet of salvation – 26, 33, 58
helper – 18, 94
herd mentality – 90
high blood pressure – 12, 16, 44, 100, 119
high-calorie – 48, 129
Hippocrates – 120
Hollywood – 36
hopelessness – 45, 50
hydrogenated oils – 119
idol – 36, 67
ignorance – 90
imagination – 35, 36, 42, 58, 71, 73, 74, 77, 94, 100, 150
immune system – 43, 68, 75, 78, 97, 107
imperfections – 27, 59, 65

impulsive actions – 45
indicator – 45, 91, 138
indigestion – 45
industrialized farming – 114
inferior gods – 33
inheritance – 92, 145
insecticides – 97
instinct – 31, 33, 36, 37, 139
intelligence – 18, 28, 32, 33, 34, 43, 52, 83, 90, 123, 147
intentional about life – 6, 149
intercessory prayers – 76
interdependencies – 61,
internal conversation – 42
intervention – 13, 45, 54, 66
intimidating – 69
James F. Balch – 80, 99
James Forbes – 133, 134
Jehovah – 68, 70
John Cherry – 104
journal – 76, 78, 103, 105
joy – 19, 24, 27, 34, 49, 57, 75, 92, 94, 147, 150, 151
juice fast – 134
Kingdom of God – 20, 21, 31, 35, 60, 65, 73, 90, 93, 95, 99, 108, 119
kitchen – 63, 100, 102, 103, 104, 134
kosher meats – 121
lack of concentration – 45
lack of time – 12
Larry Lea – 65, 91
Larry Wood – 49
leadership training – 63
leftovers – 139
legacy – 143
less is best – 120, 126, 129, 131
life force – 21
life of prayer – 69, 81, 149
live well – 17, 36, 46, 56, 69, 70, 86, 93, 142, 147, 148
living will – 145
loneliness – 45
love as belief system – 16
love at church – 64
love God – 20, 21, 40, 54-57, 82, 84, 88, 113
love others – 55-57, 60, 61, 67
love self – 54, 67
loving family – 61, 65, 66
low self-esteem – 45
low-brain thinking – 36
lunch – 106, 139, 152, 153, 156
M.R. DeHaan – 72, 121
magnesium – 130, 132
maintenance – 96, 105
Marl Stengler – 80
Mayo Clinic – 43, 132
meals – 46, 63, 114, 120, 126, 129
meat – 6, 46, 84, 99, 116, 117, 120-122, 125, 126, 128-132, 134, 139
meatless meals – 129
medicine – 7, 10, 11, 46, 48, 78, 97, 116, 117, 120, 140, 149
meditation – 62, 73, 75
meekness – 49
memory loss – 45
mental disorder – 40, 41
mental health – 33, 39-42
Michael Van Straten – 115

micronutrients – 45
mind's habit – 31
mindless eating – 101, 109, 123
mindless response – 37
minerals – 45, 118, 128, 132, 138
miserable – 39, 143, 146
missionaries – 126
modern medicine – 46, 48
monetary costs – 52
motivating factor – 58, 108, 146
motivation – 83, 112, 113, 146, 147
National Cancer Institute – 121
National Health and Nutrition Examination – 137
National Institute of Health – 129
National Sleep Foundation – 77
negativity – 34, 47
neighbor – 55, 61, 76
nervous system – 46, 133
new creature – 21
newborn – 58
nightshade – 130
non-food – 131
nourish – 42, 48, 59, 71, 81, 95, 102, 114, 123, 124, 137, 140
nutrients – 41, 43, 45, 46, 115, 117, 118, 121, 123, 124, 133
nutritional deserts
nuts – 46, 125-128, 131, 140
obedience – 22, 27, 28, 34, 36, 52, 54, 57, 59, 65, 70, 84, 92, 109, 114, 122, 139, 141-143
obesity – 46, 78, 119, 131, 135
obsession with self – 57
obey – 28, 52, 65, 67, 86
one-of-a-kind – 57, 146, 147
one-way conversation – 71
organization – 96, 104
organizations – 13, 64, 90, 145
original diet – 117, 118, 120, 124, 126, 140, 141, 149
overeating – 46, 47, 132
overstimulation – 103
oxygen – 56, 103, 110, 137, 150
pain – 11, 19, 40, 45, 48, 50, 51, 53, 58, 92, 100, 107, 116, 138, 145
pasteurized – 117, 118
patience – 49, 84, 94, 141
Paul Pitchford – 130
perfect – 25, 36, 41, 46, 50, 60, 61, 64, 65, 66, 79, 83, 120, 150
perfectly imperfect – 60
preserved – 63, 120
personal trinity – 15, 93
pesticide residues – 116
Pete McWilliams – 34
Pew Research Center – 101
pharmaceutical – 13, 14, 41, 116
physical exertion – 90
plant protein – 130,
plant-based – 117, 118, 121, 126, 127, 130
P.M. Smith – 65
political nature – 64
pollutants – 97
poor eating – 41, 46, 48, 106
poor posture – 45
popular culture – 11, 13, 92
pornography – 35, 37
poverty – 35, 92, 132

prayer framework – 70, 71, 76, 77, 80, 81, 105, 149

prayer life – 45, 66, 69, 70, 76, 81, 91, 96, 114, 149

prayer partner – 79, 80, 112

prayers for others – 76

prayers of thanksgiving – 76

prevention – 13, 74, 89, 129, 138

primary care – 6, 53-56, 58, 60, 66, 67, 68, 146, 149

Primary Caregiver – 68

priority – 6, 67, 140

privilege – 50, 68, 71, 73

proclamations – 93

procreate – 37

productive – 50, 69, 91, 123

profile of a well person – 53

promiscuity – 37, 47

promises – 26, 27, 56, 66, 72, 75, 80, 82, 135, 142, 147

promotion – 142-145

protective awareness – 75

protector – 18, 33, 94, 99, 119

protein – 46, 118, 121, 125, 126, 128, 130, 132, 137

public policy – 13

purchasing power – 13

pure is sure – 126, 135

purpose, living on – 6, 19, 83

raw milk – 116, 117

realign – 53

rebellion – 50, 92

recharge – 91, 106

red meat – 46, 125, 128

reflection – 16, 24, 29, 32, 38, 43, 47, 64, 66, 68, 95

rehydrate -- 63

relationship hopping – 45

relationships – 12, 19, 24, 32, 35, 37, 39, 41, 42, 45, 57, 59, 65, 87, 88, 90, 105, 115

relationship with God – 9, 16, 19-21, 27, 29, 60, 61, 64, 65, 72, 89, 94, 146

release – 58, 74, 85, 150

renewal – 73, 74, 95, 99, 112

renewed mind – 24, 27, 72, 112

reserves – 38

resources – 6, 13, 16, 18, 23, 45, 53, 70, 72, 91, 106

respect – 44, 59, 64, 65, 101

rest – 38, 53, 59, 73, 77, 79, 94, 95, 100, 102, 103, 106, 144

reverse – 15, 50, 117

Richard Foster – 43

righteousness – 26, 27, 35, 61, 79

ringing in the ears – 45

risk factors – 41, 44

road rage – 44, 45

sacred place – 54, 93, 95, 105, 135, 149

sacred vessel – 47

sacrificial death – 65

salt – 115, 121, 129, 130, 133,

salt of the earth – 30

salvation – 26, 27, 33, 58

Satan – 18, 21, 23-25, 70, 116, 122

Savior – 21, 25, 34, 51, 61, 86

schedules – 95, 112

schools – 61

seasons – 39, 40, 100, 112

seclusion – 45

sedentary – 109

self-destruct – 25, 46, 81, 147

self-education – 90

self-hate – 25, 34

self-healing – 43, 46, 118, 122

self-worth – 60

sexual – 47

shame – 58

shellfish – 125, 126, 128, 129, 130

shield of faith – 26, 28

sickness – 11, 12, 16, 21, 24, 30, 46, 49, 73, 121, 138, 143

sin – 19, 47, 48, 49, 56, 72, 119, 150

sleep – 23, 29, 45, 46, 47, 48, 52, 54, 76-79, 94, 97, 101-104, 108, 111, 132, 152, 153

sleep deprivation – 48, 78, 102

sleep hygiene – 77, 102

smoking – 39, 89, 151

social media – 12

soldiers – 10, 31, 46, 91, 92, 93, 99, 110, 114, 143, 144

spiritually nourished – 71

spiritual compass – 24

spiritual creatures -- 50

spiritual death -- 18

spiritual signs -- 45

spirulina – 128, 134

standard of care – 58

staying in the moment – 42

stewards – 6, 9, 15, 52, 77, 84, 108, 114, 144, 145

stress – 26, 27, 32, 37-41, 43-45, 48, 64, 67, 74, 75, 76, 80, 87, 104, 105, 106, 111, 139, 147

stretching – 73, 75, 111

substance abuse – 41, 45, 47,

sugar – 44, 46, 78, 115, 118-120, 125, 126, 128-137, 140

sugar-sweetened beverages – 136

Surgeon General – 109

sustainable – 6, 13, 65, 114, 119

sweaty palms -- 45

sweeteners – 119

symbol of success – 47

systemic dysfunction – 13

T. Colin Campbell – 117

tactics of Satan – 24

techniques – 69

technology – 11, 35, 38, 48, 80, 101

television – 12, 35, 47, 77, 91, 99, 103, 104, 109, 123, 152

temperance – 49

territory – 31, 34, 88, 93, 99, 104, 133

Terry Dorian – 119, 136

theocratic – 65

time – 66-69, 71, 73, 82, 86, 91, 92, 105, 147

time log – 152, 153

time management – 42, 91

transition – 13, 31, 53, 60, 112, 124

trap – 48, 54

Trinity – 17, 18, 21

Trinity health – 24, 48

trustworthiness – 64

truth – 91, 92, 94

truth about feelings – 42

unconditional – 62

unforgivingness – 51, 58, 65, 74

unique path – 86

unique talent – 84
universities – 13
unlovable – 66
unorganized – 90
untruths – 122
upset stomach – 45
value system – 9, 42, 50, 95, 105
values – 11, 17, 24, 35, 37, 42, 94-96, 100, 102, 106
vegetables – 41, 46, 48, 79, 99, 106, 114, 116, 117, 118, 120, 121, 125, 126, 127, 128, 129, 130, 134, 137, 139, 140
violation – 32, 47
virus – 34, 78
vitamins – 7, 45, 118, 128, 132
vulnerable point – 32-36, 38, 39, 40, 44-46, 50, 51
walking in love – 60, 87
Wall Street – 36
war – 10, 11, 21, 23, 32, 52, 114
warfare – 65, 74
water – 46, 52, 53, 74, 103, 106, 116, 121, 126, 134, 136-140
weak in spirit – 50

wealth – 30, 33, 92, 121, 131
WebMD – 43
welfare of others – 61
wellness culture – 13
wellness lifestyle – 7, 15, 16, 19, 53, 94, 99, 107, 108, 147, 150
wellness path – 25, 39, 91
whole grains – 46, 48, 99, 118, 125, 126, 128, 129
whole health – 9
wiring – 19, 21, 60, 133
witness – 50, 64
Word of God – 26, 27, 31, 32, 33, 86, 98, 114, 125, 148
workaholic – 91
work-life balance – 87
World Health Organization – 40
worry – 42, 45
worship – 20, 33, 59, 65, 70, 72, 79, 94, 139
wounded – 46
wrongdoing – 19, 107
zeal – 50

God is our Creator. God is Love. God is Truth.

Acknowledgements

I am thankful for the opportunity to honor the Father.

A special thanks to my husband Herbert Jordan III for your love, leadership, and covering. You are my good and perfect gift.

Thanks to my dad, Rev. Robert T. Coleman; my mom, the late Lavenia L. Coleman; my wonderful sisters and brothers—Joyce, Gerri, Robert Jr., Tim, Bruce, and Sheila; and my entire beautiful, God-given family.

Thanks to the special people who poured into me during this project.

Thanks to Joseph and Marijane Lawson for providing the retreat to write this book.

Thanks to Darlene Andrews for your time and review of the book.

Thanks to Pastor P.M. Smith and Mrs. Delores Stanton Smith for your Christian leadership.

To my prayer partner, Fran Roach, thank you.

Thanks to the best editors Kassel Coover and Melissa Cox.

Thanks to all of the people who have touched my life.